Impatient Nation

HOW SELF-PITY, MEDICAL RELIANCE AND VICTIMHOOD ARE CRIPPLING THE HEALTH OF A NATION

Dr. Robert J. Haley

Big Mike
you had a great
wrestling career. If
you put those principals
to life you cannot
be stopped strength Health
yours in
Doc Haley

ISBN: 1492255297
ISBN 13: 9781492255291

To my loving family for their support
Mom and Dad
My brother and sister, Glen and Jennifer, and their spouses, Lisa and Andy
My niece and nephew, Megan and Aidan; may they grow up in a more patient and healthy world.

ACKNOWLEDGMENTS

There have been many people throughout my life that have provided assistance and support. And for their help through the maze of life I am grateful. In writing this book there are some people I would like to acknowledge and thank for their support in this project.

To my office staff that helped juggle the demands of running an office and my needs for writing this book.

Jen Pritzaff – office manager at Haley Chiropractic for contributing to the chapter on champions by setting her own example.

Rachael Reis – office assistant, who is now a full time photographer, for spending many hours creating the cover for this book.

Kattia Rojas – my other office assistant, who used her graphic arts skills to make my caricature, which was used on the cover.

To the McMahon Brothers, Steve, Robbie, Eddie and Kevin, who are my second family, for passionate dedication to sports and fitness and work ethic, that supports the premise of this book.

Cindy Capitani – editor, for providing her wisdom and editing skills to provide the structure of the "Impatient Nation."

Linda Rentschler –author, for providing her literary wisdom to make this process much easier.

Joe Carini- Renowned Strength Coach, for providing the forward and endorsement and for making Carini's House of Iron the strength haven it is.

Kurt Angle – Olympic Gold Medalist and Professional Wrestler for providing the information on BarnDad's Fiber DX, and dedication to help fight obesity.

Kelly Halbrock – for providing additional information and flyers for BarnDad's products.

Chris Vender and his wife Sanelia of MMA University, and MMAU Management, for their endorsements and confidence in working with their athletes.

Vanessa Porto – Woman's Pro MMA fighter, for her support and endorsement.

FOREWORD

During my years as a top powerlifter and strongman I always trained hard and set high goals. Nothing was out of reach and I pass that attitude along to the athletes I train. In working with some of the world's best athletes one thing is for sure, you have to have desire. Having that desire to succeed is a must trait whether you want to be healthier or perform at your best. If you set your goals and have a plan all is left is desire and commitment. Top athletes know what it takes to win; now it's up to you.

The choice is obvious — you want to be healthier and you need to be healthier. The problem is that too many of us make excuses. We allow ourselves to become distracted and lose focus, shifting from one diet to the next or one exercise routine to the next without any guidance. "Impatient Nation" provides that guidance. It helps set the stage for achieving your health goals. You don't have to be an elite athlete to follow this book, just someone who wants to strive higher. Read the following pages and follow the advice and with a little patience you too can be a champion.

Always remember: do more than anyone asks of you! Go to your limit and BEYOND!!!

Joe Carini

Joe Carini is a former 6X New Jersey Strongest Man and Renowned Strength Coach to numerous NFL stars.

TABLE OF CONTENTS

INTRODUCTION

On March 18, 1936 in Jersey City, N.J., Robert George Haley was born to Adolphie and Robert Haley. Throughout his life, my father did most of the right things. He served his country on the front lines of the Korean War as a Marine, he worked hard for the railroad, got married and raised three children — two chiropractors and a lawyer. Even with the fact that he was an ex-marine in tip top shape and was fairly athletic as a youth, dad developed a weight problem. I remember a moment when he took me to my first Olympic style weightlifting meet in high school. We watched as a lifter prepared to try to lift 240 pounds over his head. Dad turned to me and said "let's see if he can lift my weight," which he didn't.

Dad was around 40 years old at the time and throughout the years he ballooned to 300 pounds. No confusion about his situation, just poor eating habits and no exercise. He also smoked for most of his life and seemed to always be under stress. To his great credit he never blamed his poor health on anyone or anything but his own actions. He would always tell me, my brother and sister to take care of ourselves, and never get like him because it was terrible being unhealthy.

I did not realize it at the time, but as I became a healthcare provider and started to practice, I realized how important his words were. My dad was at least verbally taking personal responsibility for his lack of health. I grew up in an era where, in my opinion, there was much more personal responsibility for your actions, so this was not strange to me. However, this does not seem to be the case today.

I have consulted with patients that do everything you could imagine to sabotage their health. These patients also do something quite similar – they play the blame game. It is some doctor's fault, or their kids, spouse, job, parents, you name it, they will blame it. They run from doctor to doctor to get what they are looking for. It comes in the form of a diagnosis. They have sciatica, hypertension, diabetes, tendonitis, bursitis, gastritis and every other ailment under the sun.

Now if a doctor tells you that you have a medical condition, you would feel that it has to be managed medically. I mean if your car makes a rattling noise it is the mechanics problem to fix. Don't worry about all the pot holes you constantly run over. That's the city's fault, they need to fix them. However until they do it might also help to try to avoid running over them if you can. It's the same situation with your health. Most people let their doctor manage their diabetes, backache, headaches, etc. However, they conveniently forget or are unwilling to do their part, like point to the issue in your lifestyle that's contributing to the problem.

Unfortunately, my dad stopped at phase one. He took ownership of his situation but he did not get to the next level. He tried on occasion, but did not change his lifestyle and he left us too early. The most excited he ever became was when his grandson Aidan was born. Luckily he got to enjoy the little guy for about six months. He talked about things like getting him his first bike, taking him to school in the morning as he got older and watching him play sports. Dad even bought a bench so that when Aidan visited he would have a place to sit and play with his toys. Sadly, he never saw that bench be put to use.

He also never met his granddaughter, Megan. I wish I had a nickel for every time my brother and me said how much he would have loved her. She is so similar to him, it would have been great.

That is what life and health are all about. It is not about blood tests, heart rates, body compositions or push ups. These are all components of getting there, but it's about your quality of life, your longevity and the time you are around to do the things you cherish like being around to dance at your granddaughter's wedding. That is what health is all about and you have more control than you think. You can steer your own ship. It can be a smooth sail or you can hit an iceberg. The choice is up to you.

In continuing to remember my dad, when I was a kid every year or so he would sit at the kitchen table and read a small, thick book. This book had to do with his work on the railroad. He would do this for a few weeks at a time. It was the only time I would see him really read something. This was the complete opposite of my mom who was always reading. He would be real intense with his study and once I asked him what was he reading. His eyes did not leave the page and he just said, "The Book of Rules." It was the book he needed to do his job, be safe and make it safe for others. It was his work manual and he was tested on it.

We all have used manuals to guide us through the game of life. Whether it is a railroad safety manual, cookbook or worker's policy manual, we use blueprints. This book is your blueprint. Done correctly it will make sense to you, test you and change your life. Follow this book of rules and you increase the chances of dancing at your granddaughter's wedding. So let's get to work.

PART I –
HOUSTON WE
HAVE A PROBLEM

Chapter 1

A NATION OF SICKNESS

The U.S. spends more money on health care than any other country. We also rank among the poorest when it comes to health. The World Health Report 2000 ranked the U.S. healthcare system 37th in the world. In 2006, we were ranked 36th for life expectancy while being ranked number one in healthcare spending per capita.

Why is there such a vast difference between what we spend and the state of our health? Because good health is so much more than just a matter of money – it's a matter of you. Every one of us has to ability to change our own healthcare status.

We make choices every day about how to eat, exercise and deal with stress – good choices and bad ones. At a seminar, I once heard a speaker say, "Nutrition is not really that hard. Here is an apple and here is a doughnut. Which one should you eat to be healthier?" It is more complex than that as we will see later, but his point is well taken.

Although health professionals spend numerous hours in school, pass multiple board exams and spend a tremendous amount of time and expense at postgraduate seminars, people still refuse to listen to us. It's been my experience that most people will not even take simple steps to change their lifestyle – even if it's for their own good. Sure, they might cooperate when they have an ailment. However, once they feel they have cleared the hurdles, it's back to business as usual.

Kids are growing fatter at an alarming rate, due in part to a more sedentary lifestyle made up of computers, smart phones and video games.

More than a quarter of the U.S. population is obese and that will only grow as our nation of chubby, inactive children move into adulthood. Organized sports help, but there is a dividing line between the players and the bench-warmers, the athletes and the bookworms. The spontaneous, run-out-the-door and play a game of tag type of activity is not found in too many neighborhoods today. In order for kids to get active, schedules must be drawn, play dates made and some kind of order imposed. Combine lack of movement with the habits of convenience foods and the availability of high-sugar, high-fat snacks, and the result is not hard to predict.

The Saga of Willie B

Here's a typical situation of how we deal with our health. Willie B is a 45-year-old, overweight man whose only exercise is walking a few blocks to his job from the subway. At work, Willie B sits his oversized butt in a non-ergonomically designed chair, in front of a non-ergonomically set-up computer terminal. He's been doing this Monday through Friday, six to eight hours a day, for the past 20 years. This repetitive routine is self-torture and is sadly all too common in today's society.

No one wants to live in misery. No one prays to feel worse. In Willie's case, he doesn't even feel that bad; he feels what he considers normal. The problem is that Willie's idea of normal is far from a positive one. He can get up and go to work everyday without too much problem. He can relax over the weekends, deal with his family and prepare for Monday's work week. However, let's look closer into Willie's behavior and see how it is affecting his life.

Willie is middle-aged, and as we age our bodies start to break down. Due to changes in our bones, joints and muscles, we can become shorter over time. Typically we lose about a centimeter or 0.4 inches every 10 years after 40. By the time we hit 70, we might be 1 to 3 inches shorter. In addition, men usually gain weight until about age 55; women until 65. While there might be some weight loss after that, it is usually due to muscle loss, not exactly a plus.

Although our friend Willie B is far from old at 45, his weight and lifestyle factors for the previous 20 years have to be taken into account. I was being kind when I said he was overweight—Willie is really clinically obese and has a body fat percentage of 38. (Over 32 percent is considered obese in men; over 25 percent for women.) Further, most of Willie's body fat is around his waistline, which is considered worse from a health perspective.

He's been getting regular check-ups for 10 years and although has demonstrated poor health patterns, he's had no real diagnosis and his blood work has been fine. Like many Americans, he's obese, stressed and sedentary. However, he's not presenting any obvious symptoms.

It is clear that Willie has health issues but he is sent from his doctor each year with merely a subtle warning about needing to exercise. What does Willie (and most of us) do with health report like that? Usually nothing. It's not his doctor's job to spend the hours needed to educate and motivate Willie into a healthy lifestyle. Patient-doctor interaction averages seven minutes. Unless it's a matter of imminent life and death, Willie B will not be motivated, and his doctor will not be obligated. So Willie, like most of us, carries on with his life until the inevitable – and almost expected – takes place. Willie gets a diagnosis, just like so many people eventually do at some point in middle age.

During a routine exam, his doctor finds that Willie's sugar levels are off, his blood pressure is up and his cholesterol levels are through the roof. No worries. Willie, again like so many of his peers, is prescribed an arsenal of pharmaceuticals.

Willie, though he knows he is overweight and out of shape, is perplexed by his changed state of health. He starts going over in his mind who or what is to blame. Was it the few drinks he had at a recent super bowl party? His boss, who has been working him so hard? Maybe the coffee shop has been heavy-handed with the sugar. Or maybe the government agencies that create the so-call "normal" levels are conspiring with the drug companies to keep everyone popping pills.

Willie ponders the possible culprits but never considers the obvious – himself. Never once does he take his own lifestyle choices into consideration.

An Ounce of Prevention

Knowledge of your body and its function is crucial. Your body composition is the percentage of fat, muscle and bone in the body, and it's usually expressed as a ratio of lean to fatty mass. Not all fat is bad; essential fat is crucial for your body to function properly and should be about 3 to 5 percent of total body weight in men and 8 to 12 percent in women.

There are several methods to measure body fat, each with varying levels of accuracy and cost: skinfold measures, hydrostatic weighting, bioelectrical impedance analysis (BIA), dual energy X-ray absorptiometry (DXA), air displacement plethysmography (Bod Pod) and underwater weighting.

The more accessible techniques are skinfold testing – the most practical and economic method—and BIA.

The skinfold method uses calipers to measure the thickness of a fold of your skin with its underlying layer of fat. BIA measures a small, safe electrical signal passed through the body, carried by water and fluids. Impedance is greatest in fat tissue, which contains only 10-20% water, while fat-free mass, which contains 70-75% water, allows the signal to pass much more easily. You can also purchase a home scale that measures BIA.

Self-care tests also are part of taking responsibility for your health and need to be part of your regular, preventive care routine. When a screening is done in the health field, we are usually looking for abnormalities. Whether looking for a disease process in someone's blood or a crooked spine, it is not wellness. It's a necessary strategy, however, it is not true prevention or wellness.

Also, a reality that you may not know, if you are taking any medications, you probably have an ailment. What I mean by this, is if you need medication for something long-term, you are not 100 percent healthy. Healthy people usually do not require any long-term medication. I have patients that fill out their health intake forms claiming to be in excellent health, but are taking many medications. They feel that since the medication is controlling their test numbers, they do not have the ailment.

As an example, I have had people leave off on their medical forms that they have high blood pressure, high cholesterol or other ailments, but list the medications for these ailments. I would tell them that if they stopped taking their medication without changing their lifestyle what happens? Well, the condition will probably flare-up or re-establish itself, so is it really gone? That is why people on medication freak out if they can't remember if they took their pills on a particular day.

One strong word of caution about medications. For your safety, only a medical physician, who is licensed to prescribe medications, should monitor or discontinue your medication. I know a lot of well-meaning health providers, trainers, even friends, who want to encourage people to drop their medication. However, only providers that are licensed to prescribe drugs should deal with this issue.

This does not mean that healthcare providers of different disciplines cannot co-manage a patient. However, leave the medication part up to those that are trained and licensed to do so.

All good physicians' goals should be for their patients to change their lifestyle so medications are not needed or reduced. However, that is up to your behavior. I tell my patients that your medical physician placed you on medication for a reason. If you want them to reduce or eliminate your medication, you have to give them the reason to. Change your life-style and improve your health.

Excuses Will Ruin Your Life

We all have excuses – even me. My main excuse – and one of the most common – is that I am too busy. But the funny thing about that excuse is that once a health crisis hits, we're forced to make time to lie in a hospital bed.

No doubt, lack of time is a real component of everyday life that most people can relate to. The good news is, a lot of time isn't needed when it comes to doing enough exercise to affect our health in a positive manner. While working on my master's degree in exercise science I assisted post-surgical cardiac patients as a rehabilitation intern. The exercise routines basically consisted of supervised treadmill workouts and light dumbbells. Some of the patients claimed to know the benefits of proper diet and exercise prior to their heart attacks. They had warning signs in the past and were advised to take preventive measures like regular exercise. Regardless, they failed to heed the warning and take responsibility for their health.

I see this scenario on a daily basis with my back pain patients. The spinal exercises prescribed after an injury closely mirror those used as a preventative strategy except the routine is more detailed and takes pain into consideration. Yet most people won't make a lifestyle change until there is a health crisis. Worse still? Many people revert to their old habits as soon as the crisis passes.

This is why it's so important to build exercise into your busy life. Once it is a habit, once it is ingrained as part of your regular existence, it will be the old habit you revert back to just as soon as you're well enough to do so.

Another common excuse as to why people don't pursue wellness is money. Sure, everything is easier with money. A personal trainer and chef would certainly ease the burden of self motivation and meal preparation. But when it comes to wellness and improved health, money isn't an issue at all. All of the information you need is on the internet and in books – exercise routines, nutritional guidelines, meal planning and recipes. There are websites to track your goals and forums to interact with like-minded people. You can even get reminders and motivational messages sent to your phone or email, all at no cost.

Now that we have time and money out of the way as excuses, let's look at another common justification – confusion. People claim – and often rightly so – that they are simply confused about what to do and where to start. Even if they do their homework, there's an overwhelming amount of information available. This book is a blueprint for getting started. HaleyHealth Action Steps at the end of each of the first ten chapters are designed to be the starting points of the building blocks in the wellness process. Completing the action steps will help put you in the right state of mind and set the stage for the next chapter. Each step will build on the next so that by the end, you have a solid plan in place. Part four will begin to put everything together and lead into The Blueprint for Health - *Doc Haley's Pyramid of Power.*

HaleyHealth Action Steps Chapter 1:

Be honest with yourself. Take a good look in the mirror and assess your overall health—body weight, composition, flexibility, strength and medical condition.

- Get a complete physical if it's been more than a year
- Get an assessment from a fitness professional if you're sedentary
- List any ailments you have and medications you take
- Highlight those ailments that could be lifestyle related
- Write down five words that describe how you see your current state of wellness
- Write down five words that describe how you would like your current state of wellness to be
- Begin to sculpt your goals. Examples could be: "Lose 10 percent of body weight," "Lower bad cholesterol by 10 points," or "touch my toes." Other goals might include "see my doctor for a check-up," "join a gym and have a trainer evaluate by fitness levels," "check with my chiropractor to assess my joints and range of motion."
- Set the clock. Decide when you want to achieve these goals. Goals should be monitored on a regular basis. A year-long goal, for example, should be broken down into weekly, monthly and quarterly increments. This is important not only for encouragement along the way, but for reassessment and fine-tuning.

Chapter 2

THE PITFALLS OF MODERN MEDICINE

If you fall down your stairs, you get shipped to the hospital, not the health club. Everyone mostly understands that. There are some people, however, that refuse to go to the medics, even in an obvious crisis. That is their choice and sometimes it can turn out poorly.

Now I am not saying you run to the ER for every sniffle you get, but crisis is crisis. However, on the flip side you should not expect your MD or any health provider to understand all the aspects of wellness. Nowadays doctors are so specialized that they have small areas to deal with and anything outside that range is not their domain.

A funny story happened to me when I went to an ENT with a lump on my lower neck. He evaluated my neck with great care, but when my lump's location was about two inches away from his specialty zone he said that is not his location of expertise and I would have to see someone else. And he was a top doctor in his field, but only in his limited area of specialty or location. A podiatrist will not fix your teeth and an orthopedist will not handle your cardiac issue. This is a far cry from when I was a kid and the local doc handled everything and claimed to have knowledge – for better or worse—in many areas.

But in recent years, despite the age of specialty, many general physicians are at least trying to identify lifestyle and individual habits as a culprit in underlying health issues.

Unfortunately, in today's insurance environment, providers have limited time during an office visit to discuss wellness options in detail. Their primary job is to try and fix what is broken on the surface. That's why it's important for you to be well versed regarding your own health and how lifestyle factors can play a part in maintaining what the doctor fixes.

It's Not About Being Anti-Drugs but Pro-Lifestyle

Conventional medicine – what I consider crisis care – has its place. It has helped me and many others deal with critical medical issues. What I find troubling is that providers usually end up prescribing medications for whatever the ailment is. If you are currently taking medicine or have some chronic ailment, there is no need to be ashamed. The problem is, many people accept medication as a way of life – even with side effects – and never even consider making any changes to their lifestyles.

I cringe when people refer to someone who used to be sick as now doing "fine." When someone is fine, usually that means the absence of symptoms, that the person is back to pre-sickness status. However it doesn't tell you if that person is functioning at optimal level or not.

Suppose your pre-sickness status was an overweight smoker whose biggest workout was between the couch and the refrigerator. Did your health really improve or did the crisis intervention just gloss over the reality that you're an unhealthy individual spinning a roulette wheel with your health?

As a nation, we have a false perception that doctors, hospitals and pharmaceuticals improve our health.

As Americans age and gain a few pounds, they ask for pain relief to deal with joint pain and other ailments, like it is an accepted part of the aging process. You get heavy and lazy, ache and take your medications to get through the days. Is this what we have to look forward to? Talk about the golden years or the multi-colored years from all the different colored pills the average American takes as they age.

According to the Centers for Disease Control and Prevention (CDC), the use of multiple prescription drugs from 2007-2008 increased by 20% over the prior decade. The use of five or more drugs increased by 70%. During this period, half of Americans used at least one or more prescription drugs; 1 out of 10 used five or more drugs. One out of every five children used at least one or more prescription drugs. This is compared with 9 of every 10 adults that were aged 60 and over.

Joint Replacement

The senior years are becoming the titanium years with all the joint replacements performed. The medical community estimates that by 2016, around 200,000 patients that require a hip replacement and 750,000 knee replacement patients will be on waiting lists.

People assume joint replacement is part of aging; it's not. While hips and knees will wear and tear from age and stress, you can probably avoid surgery if you do the right things. Of course genetics play a role, as does how well you've been taking care of yourself through the years. But it's never too late to start on the right path, and even genetics can be overcome.

Are You Starting to Feel it's Up to You?

I have a great deal of respect for people who want to heal, whatever their specialty is. However I wanted to bring out some of the problems, which lead to an unhealthy nation within the IMPATIENT NATION.

You have to be the one to take charge of your health — not your doctor. You have to make the lifestyle changes that will allow your doctor to experience rare results: the reduction or elimination of medication, reversal of bad blood work, reversal of abnormalities. This has to be earned. On average it is difficult, but within reach.

HaleyHealth Action Steps For Chapter 2:

- When you visit your doctor or are visiting multiple doctors for opinions on a procedure do the following:

Do not clam up at the doctor: Ask questions and don't just nod your head. The more data a health provider has the better the chances of getting the proper diagnosis and treatment.

Try to have the important information bulleted. Try to be prepared and try not to ramble. If you get stomach pain when eating a certain food it may not be important that they switched your cable channels or something. Believe me people ramble.

- Keep an updated list of all medications past and present, OTC, supplements. Once again, the more data the better.

- Keep results of any test and procedures that you have had. Know what these results and procedures mean to your health. The more informed you are the better you can manage your health.
- Find out your options for treatment, surgery, etc. Remember every procedure has risks.
- If you opt for surgery know what the procedure will entail, recovery, risks, etc.

Chapter 3

THE RIGHT OF HEALTH

This is the chapter that I like the best. It is the part of the book that grasps the concept of the IMPATIENT NATION to the tee. But first let me go over my background so you can understand who you're dealing with, how I view things and how I come to my conclusions. I am a product of the 1970s as I was born in 1961 and hit my teenage years in the mid-70s. In my opinion, people were grittier than they are today. This was before everything had to be politically correct. If you got in trouble in school the French justice system was applied. Or at least what we thought they did in France. This meant you were guilty until proven innocent.

You were expected to love your family, faith and country. I know there was a lot of protest and anti this and anti that but still people seemed more close knit. Most of us grew up with a sense of pride and toughness. And one other thing we grew up with was (pardon my French) "BALLS." This meant if you had an issue the first order was to try to fix it yourself. And if you could not fix it you sheepishly would ask your friends and family for help. But you developed personal responsibility.

It's All About Personal Responsibility

Without personal responsibility you are leaving your health in the hands of others. This is not wise nor is it beneficial. Neither is leaving everything up to you. When you have personal responsibility you take care of your end and if needed, someone qualified will take care of their end.

This does not happen as much as it should, as in my opinion most folks feel that they are entitled. They feel that the rules do not apply to them. They will do whatever they please and someone else must pick up the pieces. You see them at parties or at ball games or walking down the street. Self-abusing people not caring about the pending health crisis that will most likely fall on them. Instead it is think about today and let others worry about me tomorrow.

Self-control and discipline are key components to personal growth. Without them, you can develop certain personality traits that can lead to people failing to take responsibility for their health. When this happens, those type of people believe they can abuse themselves and someone else is responsible for the bill. They present themselves to healthcare offices across the country and just want a quick fix. If they are obese or have some ailment, it is never their fault. They blame doctors, medications, treatments or whatever. They complain about how some provider did not help them and the hospital staff was rude. It is never their fault.

You Need a Certain Level of Self Control to be Healthy

Now in reviewing un-controlled actions of people it reminds me of this. You have to have a level of self control to succeed in being healthy. It takes a level of discipline, patience and desire. There are countless numbers of people that decide this is it. They are getting in shape and they will start to turn their life around. And to these people I salute the thought and effort. However, many of these gung ho warriors fall by the wayside once a crisis happens. This crisis could be something as benign as a dinner party in which they indulge a little or it can be something stressful that makes them fall off the wagon.

This is an important crossroad – crisis reaction. Some people will lose their momentum temporarily and get right back on track. For others, a slip-up can be a total derailment back to victimhood.

If you are not taking care of yourself you are bartering with your health every day.

Health Care versus Crisis Care

One of the reasons for what I call an "entitlement mentality" could be our viewpoint on health insurance. Health insurance and health care, in dissected terms, really mean crisis insurance and crisis care. I made this designation earlier but I realize it can be confusing. Let me try to clarify this situation so we are all on the same page. When you see the words health insurance or healthcare being used, I want you to quickly replace the word health with crisis. Because for the most part that is what it is used for and what it really means.

I do not think this is done to deceive anyone. It seems to sound better to use the word "health" as opposed to "crisis." It is more polite to call someone "stocky" as opposed to "obese," or "thrifty" as opposed to "dirt cheap." Now I know some will argue about preventive services being offered in our healthcare system. Most of these services are to screen or prevent a crisis from occurring. This is extremely important and very necessary for early detections and survival. However, unless you address the cause of the problem it will always be a major issue. True health status will not change and we will keep putting out fires after the building has burned. How about we not play with matches?

Let's try to compare your health coverage with your auto coverage. When I last looked, in my state you have to have auto insurance if you drive a car. Now I am against forcing people to buy health coverage. In my opinion, it dilutes your rights. It is your body and up to you to take care of it if you please. However, you need to understand the risk you are taking. And if enough of you ignore the health risks of your lifestyle that means increased insurance premiums for all.

Let's get back to auto insurance coverage for a minute. Does your auto coverage pay you for your oil checks, tune ups or general car maintenance? NO? It is for car crisis care in the unfortunate event you have an accident, which is a CRISIS. Sounds like most health coverage plans.

I once underwent a preventive screen to see if I had a major problem brewing. As it was determined that I did not, I was sent home with no answer or evaluation of why my body was responding the way it was. Structurally I was cleared until my situation presented itself with more concrete evidence of pathology. At that point, a doctor or tech can say eureka I found something, you've got mail or it's all bad.

Now understand these tests are necessary and I want more things covered under insurance plans. Unfortunately the way healthcare, (remember to switch to crisis care), is going in the future it might cover less if you have more regulations involved. If this happens, personal responsibility will have to rise. Your personal knowledge of how the human body works will be paramount. And more specifically the knowledge of how your body works will be crucial.

Everyone's Health is an Individual Affair

Remember everyone has different needs, and health strategies should be individualized. After practicing for over 19 years and studying health for another 13-14 years prior, and spending more than a few thousand hours in postgraduate and home study, I recently heard the best answer about health ever from a provider. As I was attending a functional blood nutrition seminar with a brilliant practitioner, he gave the audience 15 hours of golden information to improve health. During a break I asked the speaker several questions about nutrient timing or something of that nature.

After hearing him go through hours of science and specific mechanisms of how nutrition can be used to help heal the body, he gave the answer. His brilliant answer was "I don't know." The answer might sound like a cop out, but the explanation hit the nail on the head. He said that everyone is different and responds differently to different situations. To get a more precise answer you need to know the individual.

We tend to try to use guidelines and strict rules to fit everyone in mass categories, rather than look at what an individual's body is doing. He mentioned the notion that suggests that everyone has to eat breakfast to balance blood sugar. He mentioned that it works for the majority of people. He also mentioned that he never eats breakfast. He also eats a delayed lunch and has stable blood sugar. That does not make it right or wrong but it's perfect for him. I am pretty sure he did not wake up one morning and have his whole body physiology figured out. This comes from a series of self-trials and errors. This also means some failures along the way. The key is to learn from your failures and turn the experience into a positive result.

We tend to have this cookie cutter mentally in health care that one size fits all. Here is the purple pill for that ailment; if you have this, here is the blue pill; and if they don't work, here comes the white pill. People tend to do this too. They talk to friends or listen to the scuttlebutt and engage in activities without any mental prep work. Do you know how many middle aged women I saw with hip and back problems when kick boxing exercise routines became popular a few years ago? Here were people who never exercised and could barely rise themselves from a chair, begin to violently kick their legs in all different directions.

How many people I see taking some supplement that they heard of on the radio without even knowing how their biochemistry is functioning. Every program — whether exercise, nutrition, structural care, stress reduction — should be as individualized as possible, according to a person's present situation, fitness level and capabilities.

Looking Toward a More Wellness Approach

Unfortunately modern healthcare is geared at looking for disease and rarely evaluates the individual in a wellness model. The vision for healthcare in the 21st century is supposed to include a heavy emphasis on wellness, but it is still disease control oriented. And you know what? It should be heavy on disease control because there are so many diseases out there. This means many sick people and not well people, hence the IMPATIENT NATION.

Once again, it is extremely important to look for, and try to help the patient in a disease state. With the nation's population becoming more unhealthy, this approach takes up the front row. And in my opinion, due to limited insurance coverage, the true wellness model is lost in traditional healthcare.

Health Coverage Takes Stage

The beginning of health coverage in this country began with earnest roots. In the early part of the century healthcare was vastly primitive by today's standards. Prior to the 1920s medical care was sparse and patients were generally treated in their homes. Due to the basic technology of healthcare or lack of technology, medical expenses for care were relatively low. In a survey by the Bureau of Labor Statistics in 1918 it was found that in evaluating 211 families in Columbus, Ohio, only 7.6% of their annual healthcare expenditure was for hospital care. Most of the expenses from illness came from not being able to go to work.

A 1919 study by the State of Illinois showed that lost wages due to illness were four times greater than the medical expenses associated with treating the illness. With this being the case, most people did not have health insurance, as it was not a priority. In contrast, people purchased sickness insurance, which worked like a disability insurance to cover lost wages or income in case of illness.

Currently the debate continues about nationalized health care. In an earlier situation, people feeling health care insurance was unnecessary helped defeat a proposal for a national compulsory system. The American Association sponsored a proposal of this type of coverage for Labor Legislation (AALL) in several states. This proposal was defeated due to several reasons. The reasons for this were, first: At that point in time there was a low interest in the need for healthcare as I mentioned earlier.

The second reason was that doctors, pharmacists and commercial insurance companies were all against it. Doctors feared, as they do today, that government-run care would cut their fees. The pharmacists feared it because government-provided prescription drugs might undermine their business. And the insurance companies were opposed to the legislation because it would exclude them from offering burial or funeral insurance, which at the time was a large part of their business.

So what happened to increase the need for health care? At that point in our history, it was considered unnecessary and costs were contained. What happened to make the dramatic switch was progress and technology. Treatment of illness was moving from the home to the hospital. In the period of 1920 to 1930 the quality of doctors improved, hospitals began to offer better services, and medicine became widely accepted. With people moving into the city areas, there was better access to hospital and treatment centers.

Now this is not a bad thing. Having more qualified doctors and better facilities improved health care, however with progress comes cost. The committee of the cost of medical care was formed in 1927. In their studies, they found that the average American family had medical expenses of $108 in 1929, with 14% of their total bill from hospital cost. In an urban setting in 1929, families earning between $2,000 to 3,000 a year spent about $67 annually on medical bills. That figure was based on no family member needing hospital service. If that occurred the price went up to $261. And by 1934, the hospital costs for an American family rose to nearly 40% of their health care bill.

With health care cost going up, the first modern group health insurance plan was formed in 1929 by a group of teachers in Dallas, TX who contracted with Baylor Hospital. The plan included room, board and medical expenses for a monthly fee. In 1932, Blue Cross Blue Shield began to offer group health plans. Employee benefit plans began to grow in the 1940-50s, as unions negotiated for better employee benefit packages.

In the 1950s and 60s government involvement in healthcare began to grow. Social Security coverage included disability benefits for the first time in 1954. In 1965 the government created the Medicare and Medicaid programs. And today, government involvement in healthcare is poised to expand.

As I mentioned, I like the premise of health insurance. I feel it is not as bad as politicians make it sound. I think the system definitely needs some level of reform, but massive overhaul and government intervention at the presently proposed level (which is always subject to change) is ridiculous.

The Medicare Dilemma

Look at the financial shape of Medicare and see if it can handle such a burden. In a report released in 2008, the Medicare trustees announced that the Medicare Hospital Trust and Supplementary Medical Insurance Trust Fund expenditures were growing faster than the rest of the country's economy.

The report claimed that expenditures were $432 billion (it's hard for me even write such a number) in 2007. This number was 3.2% of gross domestic product (GDP) and is expected to increase approximately 11% of GDP in 75 years. Spending for Medicare and Social Security, which are the two largest government benefit programs, cost more than $1 trillion (now it really hurts to write this) in 2008. At this rate, Medicare is expected to run out of money by 2017 and social security by 2037.

Now I do not want to get too political, as there are points on both sides. At this point it is unclear what it will look like. So heaven help us, your guess is as good as mine. However, these numbers should concern every American. What can we do to thrive in the golden years?

Does Increased Health Care Costs Mean You Will Get Healthier?

Let's look at increased health care cost due to hospital stays and illness. Is there an answer? Maybe we can try to get as healthy as possible so the use of these fine doctors and hospitals are used for the crisis care that they are intended for. Ever drive passed a medical office in the winter and glimpse in the window? They are packed with depressed immune systems and not a lot of happy campers. These poor patients wait for hours to be seen by their doctor.

The funny part is that some people rarely use conventional medical services. When I was in chiropractic school, I met many students who had never been to a medical doctor. They were some of the healthiest people I ever saw. They worked and prided themselves in staying healthy. They were not just satisfied with being symptom free; they wanted their bodies to work as they were intended to.

Physicians, don't be scared; unfortunately there will always be room for you. However, it would be nice to see health care really become health care, and crisis care used only when needed. Also, more conservative care options should be explored prior to expensive and invasive procedures. Do you want people on diabetic medication their entire lives or do you want them to eat right and exercise? Back surgery? Or try chiropractic first? Anti-anxiety drugs or meditation? You can see more people for the right reason and crisis treatments can be limited.

Crisis Care Has its Place

Remember, crisis care is important and not to be neglected. However, does everyone have to be tripping over themselves to run for all these procedures? Failure to attain a healthy body weight can lead to gastric bypass, joint replacement, diabetes, and much more. Lack of physical exercise can lead to heart disease, osteoporosis, poor posture, etc. You get my point.

HaleyHealth Action Steps Chapter 3:

- List all the health concerns you had in the past year if you can remember them.

You need to place them in one of two lists: One list will be for trauma and one list will be for all others. Examples would be if you sprained your knee that would be a trauma. If you have headaches because of an auto accident, I would place that in trauma also. If you are overweight, fatigued constantly and have sinus problems, these are examples for list number two. Keep this list until you finish this book because we will help you address many of these problems just by getting healthier.

Chapter 4

WHY IT'S NOT TOTALLY YOUR FAULT

It's not really your fault; that's partially true. We have set a strong foundation for your own personal responsibility but there are factions that make it hard. You have the media or more specific TV commercials that continually push all their fast food joints on us. You have to be very strong willed not to succumb to the temptations. They tempt you with the sight of these luscious treats that the average person cannot resist. Have you seen those commercials lately? They are done so well you can almost smell the stuff coming right out of your television.

Marketing That Really Works

This type of marketing may trigger highly sensitive individuals to run out for that juicy burger. A study published in the Journal of Neuroscience, reviewed brain scans to determine the response to food images. The participants were all normal weight individuals. This was because people that are obese have "neurohormonal changes" that affect brain function according to researchers. Their brain scans were analyzed for reactions to sets of three types of images. The images were of appetizing food, bland food and unrelated images.

The researchers quizzed the participants to determine their level of susceptibility to food cues. They had the participants fast for two hours and then assessed their level of hunger. The results revealed that prior to viewing the food cues, individuals with high food sensitivity were not any hungrier than individuals with normal sensitivity.

However, after viewing food cues the higher the food sensitivity the hungrier the participants were. This concluded that the images triggered hunger in susceptible people.

Maybe that is why while you are watching television, you suddenly jump into your car for a late night food run. You may be a susceptible one they are targeting.

Just think of it realistically for a moment. It is late at night and you are in your sleeping attire on the couch. It seems like all those fast food commercials come on at that time and they mention late night service. You think they are betting on you going to bed and waking up saying I need a whopper. I think they are trying to get you dressed and on the road for a snack. I know because they got me many times.

If the food commercials are not enough to send you down the road to gluttony, what about the drug commercials? Every one of those drug commercials has some sort of happy moment involved. If it is not the claims for a new life through weight loss or the nonstop ability to mate with your partner, it's less time dealing with your menses. Did you ever see all the warning signs for these drugs at the bottom of the screen? Well next time they are on we can get you a magnifying glass to read them.

Another problem is, what is the stuff they put in our common food choices? Does it make us want to eat more? Is it that the stuff is really bad for us, or is it a combination of both? These are very interesting points. And it makes for some good investigation and some clear-cut answers.

Getting More of a Bad Thing

First let's investigate these commercials and what is the meaning behind them. This is important to know because they are everywhere we turn. You cannot watch a TV program, (which you should not be doing too much of), without seeing a vast array of the fast food and drug propaganda. You also cannot ride on the highway without seeing all those signs out there. I have to give them credit – they look good.

Those food ads that you see have one real purpose and one purpose only: TO GET YOU TO BUY THEIR PRODUCT. Many a night I would see a Wendy's or Mickey D's commercial late at night and get dressed and run out for a midnight snack. Many of us are susceptible to this type of behavior.

This is the American way. We love to eat and enjoy having fun. And boy those places have some tasty stuff. However, overindulgence will lead to an unhealthy status and if we want to be healthy, self-control is needed. And those ads are no help if you want to be healthy.

The Influence of Marketing on Children

An interesting study was done on this subject. In this study, 118 children between the ages of 7 to 11 were showed a cartoon that had four commercials breaks. The groups were randomly assigned to either a group that viewed four food commercials or a group that viewed four non-food commercials. The group which viewed the food commercials, were watching commercials that were all for unhealthy foods like sugary cereals and potato chips.

During the study, while watching the cartoons and commercials each group's children had a bowl of gold fish cracker snacks in front of them. They were instructed to snack as they wished during the show. The conclusion of the study was amazing. The group that were watching the cartoon with the food ads, just like your kids at home do, ate a whopping 45% more goldfish crackers than the group that watched the non-food ads.

Don't Forget About the Adults

There also appears to be a similar link to the same behavior in adults. A second study published in *Health Psychology* was also done by Dr. Jennifer Harris and a group from Yale University. In this study the group looked at 98 college students aged 18 to 24. An added component to this study was that they measured students that were actually dieting. Being on a diet was figured to make temptations of food hard to resist. A few other different components were that subjects did not watch cartoons but a comedy show. Also, they did not have snacks in front of them but were presented the goodies afterwards.

The subjects were placed in three groups. One group viewed snack food ads, the second viewed nutritional food ads and the third viewed non-food ads. After they viewed the show they were told there was another study being done. This required them to taste and rate certain snack foods. The snacks varied from vegetables, multigrain chips, cookies, snack mix and trail mix. They were told to taste each snack in any amount they wanted.

Harris again found evidence that ads work. The group exposed to snack ads ate significantly more than the other two groups. Another observation: the two biggest offenders of overeating when exposed to snack ads were dieters and men. Both population segments ate an average of one third more than the other groups.

Link Between Children and Television

More evidence of this type of behavior was seen by researchers at the Harvard School of Public Health (HSPH) and Children's Hospital in Boston. They found that children who spend a lot of time in front of the television end up eating more advertised food that is high in calories and low in nutrition.

Jean Wiecha, a senior research scientist at the Harvard School of Public Health, and her colleagues looked at baseline data on dietary patterns and the television viewing habits of 548 children from the Boston area. The children were in the sixth and seventh grades. Measurements were taken 19 months later. The researchers asked the children about the snacks and beverages they viewed on television, and the amount of time they spent watching television.

The results of this research demonstrated that for every one hour increase of television watched over the baseline was associated with an additional 167 calories. That is just about equal to a soda or a small amount of snacks. Each extra hour also was associated with the snack foods that were commonly advertised. This also was connected to over consumption of sugary drinks.

They Even Got the Family Docs

Fueling this problem, well maybe not fueling it but putting an interesting twist on this, is the AAFP. The American Academy of Family Physicians was widely criticized for accepting money from Coca Cola. This obviously brought on much condemnation from health advocates.

This behavior from physicians should not surprise people that were around in the late 1940s and early 1950s. If you look on YouTube, you can still see videos of an old cigarette commercial that featured doctors being surveyed about their favorite cigarettes. Looking at this old commercial, it is humorous to see the family doctor leaving his house to tend to patients, and after a hard night's work, sit there and light up a cigarette.

That still happens today and unfortunately much worst probably happens. Individuals no matter how educated or what they are supposed to symbolize still have weaknesses. We would be foolish thinking everyone practices what they preach. At least we do not see them on commercials endorsing it.

Are Ads Improving?

Luckily, there might be a bit of a good turn in the unhealthy ad department. As least as it deals with kids, an analysis of television rating in 2003, 2005 and 2007 showed that children 2-5 years of age saw 21.9%. to 41.0% less ads for cereals, soft drinks, snacks and candy by 2007.

Similar findings were seen in the same ads in the age groups for 6-11 and 12-17 year olds. As they looked at older groups this positive trend diminished. This research was reported in the Archives of Pediatric and Adolescent Medicine.

These positive changes came about with some good old fashion pressure. The Council of Better Business Bureaus started a campaign in 2006 against the marketing of foods directly to kids. For their efforts, 19 major companies pledged to create healthier marketing plans. Coca-Cola and three large candy companies said they would stop advertising directing to kids under 12.

To monitor the progress of these programs, Nielson Ratings data on children's TV viewing behavior in 2003, 2005 and 2007 was analyzed. By 2007, children ages 2-5 saw 1.04% less drink ads. There was a regular soft drink ad decline of -68.2%, for fruit drinks, -75.0% and milk -56%. There was an increase in ads for diet soft drinks, 72%, yogurt drinks, 77.8%, and bottled water, 375.5%.

However, in the area of fast food there is a problem. The ads for these foods, which we mentioned earlier to be a real problem, rose.

There was a 4.7% increase of these ads in the 2-5 age group. There was an increase of 12.2% in the 6-11 age group and 20.4% increase in the 12-17 age group.

The researchers found more unhappy news as they monitored the corporate pledges to stop marketing unhealthy food to children. In a 2008 study they found an estimated whopping 90% of the foods that were advertised on Saturday morning children shows were junk food. As I must say, this was probably the same while I was growing up and it worked.

Not Much Has Changed Since I Was a Kid

I remember how much I enjoyed those Saturday morning cartoons. The Roadrunner and Wily Coyote and those kid's shows like the Monkees and Lancelot Link the secret chimp really caught my attention. But almost at equal value were all those great commercials.

What a great marketing tool, to advertise kid's foods and drinks during shows that were actually being watched by kids. The genius of it was profound. You offer great shows that kids have to watch every Saturday morning or they will drive their parents crazy. I watched these shows with my younger brother and sister without our parents. Usually, my dad was working and mom was doing housework. But little did they know that our young, little minds were being brainwashed with all kinds sugary, fatty junk food. Our parents did not have a chance as all three of us nagged them for the same junk food.

Remember the prizes you used to get for buying the stuff? I remember how excited I was when I had enough box tops to get a model plane from the back of a cereal box. This is marketing brilliance and they got all of us. They got me, my brother and even my sister. And they also got my neighborhood as every kid watched those shows and had their parents buy those products.

Sadly, what my siblings and I got besides the joy of watching and munching was obesity. Well maybe not obesity but we were all overweight. We also were very active in sports and we still were overweight when we were young. That is an important point to remember as we progress in this book. You have to combine solid nutrition with proper exercise if you want to be fit and healthy.

The Power of Protein

Protein and amino acids are necessary for the formation, maintenance, replacement and repair of structural components, transport systems and control mechanisms of the human body. To downplay their importance in the diet could lead to unhealthy situations down the road.

Not so Fat

The limitation of saturated fats and cholesterol seem on the surface to be the right thing to do, however these are important for health, and the phobia towards these fats prey on the nutritionally uneducated. The limitations that have been placed on consuming dietary fats and cholesterol are based on the notion that these lipid components will increase your blood cholesterol. With high blood cholesterol, the risk of cardiovascular disease increases. The problem with trying to simply just connect these factors are that consuming dietary cholesterol is not as significant a factor in elevating blood cholesterol as you may think.

Studies have indicated that there is not a strong connection between the intake of saturated fat and the increased risk of coronary heart disease. Also, data does not support connections between the intake of total fat, cholesterol, or specific fats and stroke risk in men.

Dietary fat will not make the body fat, unless it is in the presence of excess insulin. Increasing your insulin level happens when you consume foods containing high glycemic carbohydrates. This is why low carb diets have been so popular in recent years. People reduced their intake of high glycemic carbs and they were able to reduce their body fat.

Saturated fats can provide beneficial effects in your biochemistry and physiology. When you try to restrict your saturated fat intake you can affect the function of your gallbladder and decrease the absorption of fat-soluble nutrients. I am not saying to go out and douse everything in butter or stop trimming all that fat. However, understand the role of fats in the diet and what types are best.

All Carbs Are Not Equal

Being carbohydrate heavy has proven to be an unhealthy dietary strategy. For years we have been eating too many carbs and we have been getting fatter and fatter due to this. The typical American diet is way too carb heavy and the type of carbs we eat are the wrong type.

As I mentioned before, eating higher glycemic carbohydrates will elevate your insulin response and increase your body fat. In the 1980s when eating fat free was the craze, people still got fat due to all the heavy carbohydrates they were consuming. But excuse me the cookies said "fat free."

Nutritional Labels Can be Inaccurate

If this is not enough to feel like there is some kind of conspiracy against your health, here comes more craziness. There is some evidence that the nutritional facts labels can have some inaccuracies. I have four nutrition credentials and I need all of them to be able to read food and supplement labels with some degree of accuracy.

"Good Morning America" analyzed the labeled ingredients of a dozen packaged foods and found that three products contained more than 20% of what was listed on their label. Before you get too mad, the U.S. government allows for that 20% discrepancy before they will act.

So in knowing this, all 12 products were over the listed amount for at least one of its ingredients. Now in fairness to the companies, the study was small, looking at one sample of each of the products. In contrast, the FDA will look at the labels of many samples from different lots. Either way it does raise some eyebrows as to what is in your food.

Don't Skimp on the Good Stuff

Another disturbing trend is that some food makers actually skimp on their ingredients. Some examples: a chocolate manufacturer substituted vegetable oil for cocoa butter; a spice company swapped a more expensive Mediterranean oregano with one from Mexican. That's unacceptable. Give me what I pay for, whether it is good or bad, and be accurate.

Run from these to be Healthy

In talking about ingredients we need to have some knowledge about what is really bad for us. There are a number of harmful ingredients and preservatives that can cause us problems. However, there are four that should be avoided or at least very limited in our diet: trans fats, refined grains, excess salt and high fructose corn syrup. In my opinion, trans fats and high fructose corn syrup should be avoided like the plague. Refined grains and excess salt should follow this closely. The sad part is that these four unhealthy ingredients load the typical American diet. They are all around us like the air and most of us do not even have a clue of their harming ways.

Trans Fat is No Friend to Your Arteries

First let's hit on trans fats. You heard of these. A few years ago there was some kind of media hype on this topic. Trans fats are unhealthier than saturated fats and wreak havoc on your arteries. They increase your level of bad cholesterol (LDL) and decrease the level of good cholesterol (HDL). By reducing your intake of trans fat you can decrease your risk of a heart attack by 53 percent. The really bad news is that they are contained in most of the foods that people love. Foods like muffins, crackers, microwave popcorn and margarine contain trans fat.

Refined grains and salt are a little tricky. We think we understand that grains are touted as good for us so what's the beef with them. Well we are not talking whole grains, but refined grains. These grains are found in cereals, bread, white rice and white pasta and can boost your risk of heart attack by up to 30%. Also refined grains can raise your cholesterol, blood pressure, and chances for insulin resistance, diabetes, and abdominal fat. On the flip side, studies show that by consuming more whole grains you can reduce your chance of a heart attack by 20-30%. However, let's not get too happy on the grain side as there are some problems with whole grains too. They can be a cause of inflammation in our bodies. We will go into this in detail later.

Hold the Salt Please

We all know that too much salt is not a good idea, but sodium is everywhere. I have not used a saltshaker in probably over thirty years, but you know who does. The cook in the back of the restaurants I frequent or the local fast food joint you stop by for a quick bite. And sodium does not have to be added to your food by the old shaker it's already in most food we eat. The hidden sodium is not too hidden if you watch your food being prepared. You have to become a salt detective and really understand labels. You also have to understand how your food is being prepared when you are eating out.

The average American consumes around 3,375 mgs of sodium on a daily basis. Sodium intake is also higher for males as compared to females. The recommendation for sodium intake is 2,400 mg daily according to the National Committee on Prevention, Detection, Evaluation, and Treatment of High Blood Pressure.

If you can limit your sodium level to around 1200 to 1500 milligrams per day you greatly reduce your chances for increased blood pressure and heart disease. In understanding these measurements, there is about 1500 milligrams contained in about three-fourths of a teaspoon of salt. Not much salt to play around with. Most American's can well exceed that limit of a daily basis.

A 2010 article, "After 50 Years Americans Still Eat Too Much Salt," claimed that despite the warnings associated with excess salt intake we have not reduced our dietary consumption of salt in 50 years. Two researchers, Adam Bernstein and Walter Willett analyzed urine samples from 26,000 people. In evaluating urine excretion they were able to measure sodium levels. This analysis gives about a 95% reliability level of what is consumed as opposed to looking at food diaries.

They found that it did not matter what year samples were taken, the subjects consumed around 3.7 grams or 3700 mgs of sodium per day. This finding was more than 1.4 grams or 1400 mgs over the teaspoon a day recommended, and double as much for someone with high blood pressure should be consuming. There were little differences between ethnicity or age levels. Men did have a higher sodium level than women. This was explained by the higher caloric intake of the male subjects as opposed to the women subjects.

Sodium and Blood Pressure – Careful with Those Processed Meats

Americans today eat much more processed meats than in past years. Also a majority of sodium is added in the manufacturing and processing of our food. With these factors influencing our sodium intake you would think that intake would be higher today. However, researchers found that sodium levels have remained fairly stable for the last 50 years. This leads them to conclude that the increase in calories eaten on a daily basis, which leads to obesity, may be more important in the prevalence of high blood pressure than sodium intake. However, they do point out that there are major studies that show higher sodium intake raises blood pressure and hypertension risk, and can chronically elevate blood pressure. The Institute of Medicine states that high blood pressure is a "neglected disease" that costs the U.S. health system $73 billion a year.

The High Fructose Corn Syrup Saga

Sixty-three pounds. That is the number of high fructose corn syrup that the average person consumes in a year if they regularly drink soft drinks and eat sweets. High fructose corn syrup is attractive to food manufacturers because it is cheaper and sweeter than traditional sweeteners.

Research has shown this sweetener raises your heart attack risk, upsets your metabolism and can encourage overeating. It also has been shown to force the liver to pump triglycerides into your bloodstream. High fructose corn syrup can also reduce your body's chromium reserves. This is important because chromium helps you maintain healthy levels of cholesterol, insulin and sugar.

Drug Ads Can be Tricky

I hope you did not think that I forgot about the drug companies. In my research I came across a few interesting articles that shed some light. I mentioned problems with health care and prescription drugs previously, but I am not anti-drug as I also mentioned earlier. That would be hypocritical of me, as I grew up with the conventional medical approach, which is a drug for an ailment.

As a youth, I had the fluoride tablets that mottled my teeth and had my tonsils yanked out. As I became schooled about a more natural approach to health, I went about ten years without even taking an aspirin. But, as I let my lifestyle slip, my health went down. We all slip, but winners get back up and clean up their act.

That being said, if drugs are needed, they should be prescribed properly for crisis. Every physician should have a goal of reducing or eliminating the patient's medication need if possible. But that is mostly up to you. However, the drug companies can be tricky.

Not all drug ads are on the up and up. The FDA sends out approximately 100 letters per year to drug companies. In these letters they demand changes to their TV, magazine and other ads. It does not stop there. In a report by the US Public Interest Group and the NJPIRG Law and Policy Center it gets ugly. In their report they claim that drug marketers make deceptive claims to both doctors and the public for around 150 different drugs. The report indicated the following points:

- 38% of the deceptive messages to doctors and the public make unsupported or misleading claims.
- 35% misrepresented the risk and side effects of drugs.
- 22% promoted unproven drug uses.

With the information provided in this chapter it is easy to see that there are certain factions that will stop at nothing to get you to use their products. So let the buyers beware.

HaleyHealth Action Steps Chapter 4
- Cut down on watching television – you and your kids
- Substitute TV watching with healthy activities
- Learn how to read labels and avoid with the big 4: Trans fat, refined grains, sodium and high fructose corn syrup
- Review your drugs

At this point you are a rookie with this book and might not have begun to get healthy. If you are taking medications, get healthy and work with your doctor to reduce/eliminate them.

PART II –
GET READY TO
RUMBLE

Chapter 5

CHAMPIONS

In life there are winners and losers, and although there are usually shades of grey in most situations, most people would rather be closer to the winning than the losing side. You go on a job interview to get the position, you propose to your girlfriend hoping the answer is not get lost and you buy a lottery ticket hoping to hit the jackpot. You get my point.

When we deal with health, I see three main categories with some shades of grey in between. Most people I see fall into three categories: Victims, Winners or Champions, and many times, it's a lot about attitude.

If you look at the standard Webster's Dictionary, definitions of these categories can help you better equate them to your ability to be healthy. Well maybe you need some coaching, but let's first evaluate the term: Victim.

Let's Define Victim

According to Webster's, some meanings for the term victim are: an unfortunate person who suffers from some adverse circumstance, a person who is tricked or swindled, a person or thing destroyed or sacrificed in the pursuit of an object, or in gratification of a passion and one who is duped, or cheated.

If you evaluate the words in these definitions you see the magic words to victimhood. Words like "unfortunate," "suffers," "destroyed," "duped" or "cheated" resonate from people who enjoy playing the victim. "Self-pity is easily the most destructive of the non-pharmaceutical narcotics; it is addictive, gives momentary pleasure and separates the victim from reality," as quoted by John W. Gardner.

I relate the term "victim" in health care not as a poor victim of an accident or some unfortunate health circumstances. We all can understand that type of victim situation. No. I just use the term as in victim mentality.

These are the people who are not willing to help themselves. They refuse to take any advice. They believe all their ailments are the fault of others. They have all the names down to a science. The tendonitis, bursitis, arthritis and all the afflictions that accompany them. They love to talk about their complaints, but do little self help to remedy them.

Are You a Winner?

Now let's look at the other side. Let's evaluate some of the definitions for the term "winner" as it is mentioned in Webster's: the contestant who wins the contest, a person with a record of successes and one who wins, or gains by success in competition, contest or gaming.

Now as we look at the terms in this definition we can clearly sense a different tone. Words that stand out are, obviously, "one who wins or gains by success." These are more than just words, they relate to an attitude. A winning attitude is a common saying used in sports. It can also be used in everyday life. You can have a winning attitude with your job, family and yes, your health.

There Can be Only One Champion – You

In looking at the word "champion" you can see why some people become champions of their health. In reality, health has many variables. Some of these you can control and many you cannot. But a champion overcomes obstacles and strives to be the best. That is the key – strive to be your best and you can become a champion.

Look at the movie *Rudy*. His goal was to play for the Notre Dame Fighting Irish football team. This appeared to be an unrealistic goal for him. He was not the best student or athlete. Yet his goal was to become a student/athlete at one of the nation's top academic and athletic institution. He really did not have much of a plan, but he was determined.

With the heart of a lion or a "Fighting Irish" he reached his goal. He did not become a regular player or an All American; his goal was more realistic. The same applies to you. You do not have to make the Olympic team or run a marathon if it is not in the cards. Your goal should be to become more fit and healthier than you have been in the past. That is the heart of a champion.

In looking at the term champion it can be used in many ways but we all know what it implies: someone who has won first place in a competition, someone who fights for a cause, protects or fights for as a champion, being excellent, fine, splendid, superb or super and being triumphant or victorious.

The part of the definition I like best for champion is "triumphant or victorious." This explains clearly what is meant to be a champion.

Are There More Victims Than Champions?

The problem as I see it, as to why there is more of a victim mentality in society, as compared to the winning attitude of a champion, is two-fold. First, I feel that many people have never experienced the feeling of a truly earned victory. Whether in sports or in life, victory is hard to achieve for many. I often say, "You have to have been hit to know if you can take a punch."

In sticking with that premise, you have to experience winning to know how to win. If you go through life with failure after failure, it becomes easy to get frustrated and depressed, and you give up on trying to win. The key is to win your battles one step at a time and build on each success.

The second problem, as I see it, is that experiencing so much negativity puts you in the opposite mindset. You blame everything but yourself. The whole world is against you and in your mind it actually is. This becomes a dangerous cycle that is hard to break. But it can be broken if you have the patience and some guidance.

The sad part is that too many of us are on the wrong side of the fence. The funny thing is that most feel they are OK as far as their health is concerned. I have met many people who have no clue of what it means to be healthy. They are put in a weird situation as they age. As young bucks they are rarely sick and can function for the most part without any major problems. But as you know, the problems occur.

First, problems occur very subtly and then become more pronounced. For most this is like entering a strange and foreign territory. This territory usually winds up being co-managed with your physician. It will probably begin with some medications. If you don't change your habits, then more medications, and then testing is ordered. Tests are continued until probably surgery. The end point is death.

If you do not think that is true, just look out the car window when you are driving through your town. But keep your eyes on the road, no accidents please. See what is walking around, (sometimes just barely), in your community.

Don't Underestimate Your Health Situation

I have seen patients that did just a little bit of work to try to get healthy, and felt that was enough and they were just fine. One patient of mine was very inactive and about 25 pounds overweight. She claimed that she just needed to drop 10 pounds and she would be happy. Now 10 is not 25 if my math is correct, but it is a definite improvement. Well she actually lost about 10 or 15 pounds, felt great and had a better blood profile. However, like so many before her, the weight was regained and the ailments started again. Maybe she shot too low on her goals and did not fully understand what she needed to do to succeed.

Another patient was in the same boat. This patient was very inactive and grossly overweight. I asked if he had any health issues like high blood pressure or diabetes, etc. He claimed no, as he was given a clean bill of health from his doctor. So I asked if he was taking any medications. He was taking medications for high blood pressure and high cholesterol. I asked why he never mentioned these conditions. He replied that he did not have them. I asked him why he was on medications for these ailments. And as many people sadly think, the problems are gone because of the medications.

I asked him what he thought would happen if he went off the medications without changing his lifestyle. He still did not get it, so I asked how his last blood work-up results were. He said it was fine, so I asked him for a copy. Here is the interesting part. When I looked at his blood work, about 80% of the panel numbers were close to being lab or pathologically high despite his being on medication. He did not realize that technically his blood was considered lab normal, however, he was one stressful episode away from having a major health issue.

What Kind of Shape Are You in?

Let's look at some of the numbers that paint a picture on how healthy we are as a nation. On the President's Council on Physical Fitness's website, (in which, yours truly earned a patch for weightlifting many years ago) the following statistics were noted.

Heart disease is the number one cause of death in the United States. If you are physically inactive you are twice as likely to develop coronary heart disease as opposed to people that are regularly active. With that said, 37% of adults are reported to be physically inactive. Only about 3 out of 10 adults get the recommended amount of physical activity. That recommended amount of physical activity for those 18 to 64 years old is 150 minutes a week. Exercise intervals should be at least 10-minutes. We will see a shorter but more intense exercise guideline later, but this is adequate. For children and teens, the amount of activity that is recommended raises to 60 minutes a day.

Continuing on with health or lack of it, note that inactivity and poor diet can lead to being overweight or obese. Many people, however, are in some sort of denial.

People that are overweight or obese are at an increased risk for ailments such as high blood pressure, Type 2 diabetes, coronary heart disease, gallbladder disease, stroke, osteoarthritis, sleep apnea, respiratory diseases and certain types of cancers. This should at the very least allow you to pigeon hole your health concerns to at least focus on obtaining a proper weight.

More statistics indicate that 41 million Americans are estimated to be pre-diabetic. Wow, 41 million of us are heading straight toward diabetes. And probably many do not really know this is occurring. Remember, you might have normal blood lab values, however, if you do not look closer at your body's function, you can miss it. Full evaluation of functional blood values, symptom patterns and body composition is important.

This also means that most of the pre-diabetics will develop Type 2 diabetes within approximately 10 years. More than 108 million adults are either overweight or obese. This equates to roughly 3 out of 5 Americans are walking around with excess body weight.

I know I am beating this point across to you, but here is one astounding piece of information. Looking at BMI or body mass index, a level of equal or greater than 25 indicates obesity. Measuring BMI from 1999 to 2002, 65% of adults in Americans were either overweight or obese. That's 65% of Americans who have unhealthy amount of bodyweight, and thus are potentially unhealthy. This is unacceptable and has to change for us to prosper.

More Excuses Why People Will Not Exercise

What's your excuse for not achieving your optimal health? In Chapter 1 I mentioned a few, well here are a few more with my solutions:

<u>People hate or become bored with exercise</u>: The solution: Choose some type of exercise that fits you. Basically, "What do you like to do?" This can come in the form of group fitness classes, games like Wii Fit, TV fitness programs, or exercise at home. Whatever works for you, go for it.

<u>Quitting too soon</u>: Solution: you might be doing too much too soon. Remember easy does it. Treat it as a marathon, not a sprint. Another reason you might be tempted to quit is you might be confused by exercise if you are not seasoned at it. If that is the case, read and learn as much as you can to feel more comfortable. If you can, get a qualified personal trainer to help you, at least in the beginning. If exercise becomes too boring, don't quit just change it up. There are many varieties of workouts to keep you fresh. And if you are too sore or suffer an injury you have to see a good sports medicine specialist.

<u>Lack of Motivation</u>: Solution: Find the right reason to get fit and work at reaching your goal. Give yourself rewards as you reach certain goals like going out for a nice healthy dinner, or buying some new clothes for your new body. Whatever action will motivate you, just go for it.

<u>Exercise hurts</u>: Solution: you have to begin any new exercise program slow and easy. This even holds true when you are fit but are changing your current routine. Recovery is a key part to exercise and rest is

extremely important. If pain or soreness lingers you can see a good sports medicine professional for an evaluation. But do not wait; most mild soreness is usually improved in a few days and no more than a week.

Lack of Commitment and Organization: Solution: Plan your workouts in advance and start with small goals that you can fit into your schedule. You must stick to it to be successful. Make getting fit a priority. The busiest people on the planet find time to fit exercise into their daily schedule. If they can do it so can you.

Let's Get to Work

Now that there are no more excuses, let's get to work. Well it sounds easy and at least you have some strategies for success but you have to want it.

The good news is where there is a will there is a way. And if you dedicate yourself you can improve your health and live longer. Researchers looked at over 5,000 middle-aged and elderly Americans and found that individuals who engaged in moderate to high activity levels lived 1.3 to 3.7 years longer than inactive individuals.

Moderate activity level is considered walking for 30 minutes a day for five days per week. If you exercise more intensively, which is the equivalent of running for 30 minutes a day for five days, you can extend your life about 3.5 to 3.7 years.

Now I know some of you are saying, "all that work and you live maybe four years longer." Well the researchers also noted that not only does exercise help you live longer it also helps you live healthier. Your quality of life improves and isn't that the key to life, living better?

As I keep saying, it is a commitment and you have to really want to change your lifestyle to get healthier. What I often tell patients is that if what they are currently doing was the right thing, they would not be in the poor shape they are in. Many have every excuse in the book, as I just mentioned. However, the bottom line is that change has to be real.

Jen Rises to the Occasion

Here is a perfect example of what I mean. This is my own personal champion story in which I had the privilege of seeing the transformation right in front of my eyes. This is the story of my long time office manager, Jen Pritzlaff. For those who follow amateur wrestling, Jen's older brother Donny was a World Class freestyle wrestler and two-time NCAA champion. Jen was, to say the least, not as fit as her All-American brother.

Jen is 30, and was heavy her whole life. At the top she weighed close to 300 pounds and was not very healthy. In interviewing Jen, she said the main reason she was so obese was nothing uncommon: She had a poor diet and lacked the proper nutritional education needed to understand what she was doing to herself. She also was very inactive, which often goes with being obese.

She also was an emotional eater. When she was depressed or needed comfort, she would eat unhealthy foods. This is a common underlying roadblock to success. If the emotional or mental reasons aren't addressed, it is hard to stick to a plan. I think this is the reason some gastric bypass patients suffer from depression after surgery – unresolved mental and emotional issues. They changed their structure but not the mental component, so the strong desire to over eat remains. Weight loss strategies should address the mental component in some form. People don't sit home at night with a bowl of broccoli; they eat cake and ice cream.

Even though Jen knew her behavior was bad for her, and despite being around a healthcare office, she did not change. It took many years for lightning to strike and it is usually unpredictable when it does. But to Jen's credit, it did and not because of some great motivational speech or TV marketing scheme. No, Jen's motivation was just a good old fashioned reason. She was tired of always feeling sick and tired. Her health was really bad, she was constantly sick, tired, lazy and had many aches and pains.

The part I find amazing was that she made this transformation all on her own. She did not try some overhyped diet program or new heavily marketed piece of equipment. She just started with a basic plan with the most important components: Desire and Determination.

I have another little secret for you. Most of the exercise routines and equipment will help you. Some more than others, but you have to be determined and stick to them. How many people use their home exercise equipment as a coat rack? How many people jump from one quick weight loss program to the next? They are acting more like a victim than a champion.

Starting Out Simply

Jen started out simple, taking it one day at a time. She began to walk around town and reduced the amount of food she ate. Pretty simple strategy isn't it? Well, not exactly. See, we all know what to do. It is the doing it that is hard, real hard. But with this simple strategy, Jen advanced to exercise tapes and really began to fine-tune her diet. This is important because if you really want to be fit and healthy you need good muscle tone and endurance. As Jen advanced to more intense workouts, her body composition improved. That is the point. The goal should be to decrease your body fat and increase your lean muscle mass. Combine this with good cardiovascular and flexibility work and you are on your way.

Jen's quality of life has improved so much. And after the initial rough times of doing such a drastic life change, she enjoys exercise and looks forward to it. Jen's basic pointers are simple. Exercise daily. If she has a busy day she will exercise a little at night but she rarely misses. Also, she watches her diet closely from Monday to Friday, but cheats a little on the weekends. But she watches herself so she does not go overboard. Find someone or something that inspires you. Jen's friend and school-mate, Rachael, lives a healthy lifestyle and helped motivate her to success. There is a saying in sports that certain players make everyone around them play better. The same is true with achieving a goal.

Dealing with Bad Genes

Jen also felt that her weight problem could have also been related to bad genetics. We hear this a lot. Every out of shape person claims to have bad genes. Jen feels that way because her sister has good body composition and growing up, there was not much difference in exercise and eating between them. Studies show that genes can react to the environment they are placed in. If you are genetically predisposed to weight gain, it can be harder to lose weight. However, you can accomplish it if you change your lifestyle.

Jen overcame these shortcomings, lost over 100 pounds and advanced her workouts to gain more fitness. She has fewer aches and pains and is much healthier. Equally as impressive: she has stopped smoking for over a year.

To all the Champions that dared to take to plunge and succeed, I salute you. To those Victims who have not yet taken the plunge – Just go for it.

HaleyHealth Action Steps Chapter 5

- Find three to five people in your life who either inspired you or you feel is a champion. They can be successful in sports, business, family, health etc, but they must have reached a definite level of success in your mind
- Interview them on why they wanted to do what they did. Was it difficult, how did they manage and was it worth it
- Ask them their three keys to success
- Apply that information to your life

Remember, talk to three to five people and use the most common and important pieces of advice they gave you. If someone is wealthy because they hit the lottery, you might not be able to use their story, but you get the idea.

Chapter 6

ARE YOU REALLY HEALTHY?

In this chapter we will get a precursor to some of the health and fitness strategies that will be presented in Part IV of this book. First, we have to make a distinction between the terms "health" and "fitness." Someone can be physically fit and drop dead of a heart attack. On the other hand, someone can have a great health profile and get fatigued while playing with their kids. So there is a difference between the two.

Being fit or Being Healthy: Which is better?

If there is a difference between being physically fit and being healthy, which one is more important? When I was sitting in my first class for my master's degree in exercise science the professor posed an interesting question. He asked the class, "What do you think is more important nutrition or exercise?" He asked if we would be healthier if we followed a perfect diet but rarely exercised, or exercised and were really fit but ate a poor diet. Without blinking, everyone answered that the nutritional component was more important.

This is an interesting point. It shows the difference between being healthy and being fit. In my opinion we should strive to be as healthy as possible, but we should also be as fit as possible. There is a certain amount of cross over between the two. If you eat properly it will allow you to be at an ideal bodyweight. This will help you move better and feel better. If you are physically fit this should also help yourself maintain an ideal weight and a strong heart.

The Definition of Health

Before we advance further we have to get a better handle on the definitions. According to the World Health Organization (WHO) the definition of health since 1948 is "…a state of complete physical, mental and social well-being and not merely the absence of disease or infirmity." This is interesting, as you may not be sick but can have lack of health. Well let's think this over because this is an important concept. How many people feel fine and then keel over. How many people go in for a routine physical and find out they have a disease process going on.

In 1986, during the Ottawa Charter for Health Promotion, the WHO stated that health is "… A resource for everyday life, not the objective of living. Health is a positive concept emphasizing social and personal resources, as well as physical capacities." This definition concentrates more on health being a resource. I suggest that health is a resource. It is one, if not the most important resource you have and should be valued as such.

The term "health" is often used on many different fronts like, "financial health," "business health," etc. However, most people understand the term as in physical health and mental health. Physical health will address good body health, which is health from good nutrition, exercise and proper rest. Mental health refers to a person's cognitive and emotional well being. If one has good mental health they are free from mental disorders. According to WHO, mental health is "a state of well being in which the individual realizes his or her own abilities, can cope with the normal stresses of life, can work productively and fruitfully, and is able to make a contribution to his or her community."

These two aspects are important to set you in the right direction and should be maintained throughout your life. According to WHO, the following have a bigger impact on your health than access to health care: where you live, the environment, genetics, income, education level and your relationships with family and friends. Detriments, WHO reports, include: Our economy and society; where we live, what is physically around us, and what we are and what we do. The last one solidifies the premise of this book. It is the person's individual characteristics and behaviors that relates to what we are and what we do.

Understanding the Role of Fitness

You should be able to have a better understanding of what health is at this point. What about the term "fitness?" You can be "financially fit," "morally fit" and have a "fit mind," but for our purposes we are going to address physical fitness. Physical fitness is defined as "a set of attributes that people have or achieve that relates to the ability to perform physical activity" as described by the US Department of Health and Human Services.

How we measure how fit we are can vary. It depends on what aspect of fitness you are looking at. A weightlifter has a different level of fitness than a marathon runner. There are different physical demands placed on the body with different activities. When I was a wrestler, my body was put through a certain training routine and placed under certain types of stresses. Wrestling demanded more muscular endurance and cardiorespiratory capacity than when I competed in weightlifting.

In the sports of weightlifting and powerlifting, more emphasis is placed on strength and power. This is reflected in how you train. You do not see competitive weightlifters running long distances in their training routines. However, to measure the level of total physical fitness an individual possesses, we will look at five components. The five components measured are cardiorespiratory endurance, muscular strength, muscular endurance, body composition and flexibility.

If you score well on all of these components you are said to be physically fit. If you stumble on one or two of these areas then work in those areas is needed.

Your Body Has to Breath and Endure

Cardiorespiratory fitness is the ability of your body's circulatory and respiratory systems to be able to supply fuel during sustained physical activity. To increase your cardiorespiratory fitness you need to engage in activities that keep your heart rate elevated at a safe level for a sustained length of time. This can be accomplished by running, swimming, bicycling and intensive interval training.

Muscular strength is measured by the amount of force your muscles can exert during an activity. This can be achieved by strength training, which will provide the proper resistance needed. You can also increase you muscular strength by using any type of resistance from either weights or objects or going against gravity. A common mode of training I see being offered today is strongman or strongwoman training. This training is similar to the activities performed by strongman and strongwoman competitors. Many athletes will use giant tires, chains and sleds to help increase strength and muscular endurance.

Muscular endurance is measured with activities that will increase your muscle's ability to continue to perform before reaching a level of fatigue. Using strongman-type training as an example, we can break it up into these two components. In using the giant tire flip as our example, if you flip the heaviest tire you can flip once, you are measuring strength. This is similar to lifting your maximum weight in a lift for one repetition. Now take a lighter tire and flip it as many times as you can before you are too fatigued to continue. This would be a measurement of muscular endurance.

Now I know many of you are probably flipping more burgers in your backyard than tires but the example can be simplified. Let's use this scenario. We can all relate to it. Did you ever see someone try to get out of a chair by bending all over the place rather than standing straight up? As we become weaker from inactivity or age, our muscles need help. So if you lost strength in your legs and you have to use them to spring up from a chair they will fail. Due to this failure, other muscles are recruited for support and back injury can be the end result. That is lack of muscular strength. Rising from a chair should not be an endurance event, but you have to have a certain amount of lower extremity strength to rise to the top.

Now if you are doing an activity that requires lifting objects over and over like a warehouse worker, that is muscular endurance. This too can cause injury and is a common way people get injured on the job. Lifting objects repeatedly—even if they are light—will place your muscular endurance capacity in high demand. And if you are not able to handle this task, an injury can occur.

What Are You Composed Of?

This next component is very important to understand, so listen up. Your body composition is extremely important, especially when losing weight. Body composition is defined as the relative amounts of MUSCLE, fat, bone and other vital parts of your body. If you are losing weight and do not know if you are losing amble body fat, you could be losing more muscle. This can become a health problem.

Everyone Bend and Stretch Now

Flexibility is a component of fitness that I have been involved with for over 19 years. Increasing the range of motion around a joint can provide many health benefits. Once your joints begin to stiffen, movement patterns become dysfunctional. Once this faulty movement pattern happens, it can place wear and tear on the joints and lead to degeneration, AKA, arthritis. Flexibility can be achieved with exercise, basic stretching, and soft tissue and joint manipulation.

Physical Activity and Exercise Defined

I would like to make a distinction between common misconceptions. Routinely when I ask patients if they engage in an exercise routine, they claim that they get enough exercise doing housework or on the job. I realize there are many jobs that provide the necessary physical demands to the body. However there is a difference between exercise and physical activity. Physical activity is defined as movement that involves contraction of your muscles. Doing activities throughout the day, which involve movement like housework, gardening, walking, going up and down stairs, etc., are considered examples of physical activity.

In looking at exercise, it's a more specific, planned form of physical activity. It is purposeful physical activity performed with the intention of acquiring fitness or health benefits. Forms of exercise are working out, swimming, cycling, running, golfing, playing tennis and participating in sports. A good exercise program should address all components.

The real difference between the two is intensity. Most physical activity such as housework is done at a mild to moderate level of intensity. Exercise is usually monitored, and performed at a more intense level. This will help achieve an improved level of fitness. Also, if you go back to the components of fitness we just reviewed, you can see that it would be difficult to improve them with housework, gardening, walking around or similar activities.

However, I do not want to discredit the truly physical occupations that people do like heavy construction work or loading trucks. I worked my way through chiropractic school as a vender at sports venues in Atlanta. Those were very physically demanding jobs. I had to carry over 50 pounds of beer and ice up and down big steps. Between this kind of work and proper nutrition, I got in tremendous shape. However, most physical jobs will eventually wear your body down.

Sitting, however, can also wear your body down. A sedentary lifestyle can offset the exercise you do. Movement is key.

Know Where You Are – Reason for Check-Ups

Now that we understand the difference between health and fitness, and the difference between physical activity and exercise, we can begin to look at some measures. Like anything that we do that is important, we need to have a measuring point. Businesses look at profits and losses, schools look at grades, and when it comes to health and wellness, you also have numbers.

I strongly recommend my patients see their primary care physician every year to get a routine physical. There is some disagreement about the need for getting annual checks, but 12 months is a long time and a lot can change. Once you are following good wellness practices and adhering to the guidelines in this book, spreading physicals further apart is fine if your doctor agrees. However, I still like annual blood work measurements, even if you are relatively healthy. If you have issues you will probably need more medical check-ups until your problems subside. But remember: you can help your doctor and your situation by living healthier.

We will look at some important factors considered when evaluating health. Some of this advice might be different than what your current doctor evaluates. I have found that most doctors are becoming more open to expanding their diagnostic ability to help you. So if you present information to your doctor they might be cool with it. If not, find out why and you can decide the course to take. Remember, in a prevention or wellness approach, we look at physiology, structure and function rather than focusing primarily on the presence of disease. Understanding this concept is critical for health.

Specific Baseline Testing

To evaluate your health status you need to have some testing done. Here are some specific tests I recommend for males. Your doctor may order additional tests depending on your evaluation but these are a nice start.

Tests are done fasting and non-fasting; your doctor will instruct you. A lot of blood work requires a 10-12 hour fast. Once you hit the age of 40, I recommend testing every year. If you have some health issues, specific testing can be done more frequently for monitoring purposes. If you are extremely healthy as determined by your doctor, tests can be done every couple of years.

Begin with the basics like height, weight and blood pressure. As I mentioned earlier, your percentage of body fat is more important than looking at just height and weight tables. However, if you cannot get a proper body composition measurement, then a BMI will suffice.

Blood tests I recommend begin with a CBC, which stands for complete blood count. This will evaluate key factors such as red blood cells, which carry oxygen, white blood cells, which are infection fighters, and your platelet level, which are clotting particles. Looking deeper into the CBC, a hematocrit score will measure the proportions of RBC's in your total blood volume. Evaluating your hemoglobin assesses the oxygen carrying protein of the red blood cells. If these elements are low you might have some type of anemia. Further evaluation of your blood work patterns can determine if anemia is more likely a problem with iron, B12 or folic acid.

The next test recommended is a blood sugar panel. This can help you track if you are heading into the diabetic game or are still in the parking lot. I mentioned before how many Americans are becoming diabetic and pre-diabetic. These tests will help evaluate the situation. The standard measurement is the fasting glucose test. This is part of a Comprehensive Metabolic Panel. It should be paired with an A1c test, which evaluates your average blood sugar level over the prior 2-3 month period. It is recommended that if your scores are high on either of these two tests you should have an oral glucose tolerance test (OGTT).

If your fasting glucose is above 100 milligrams per deciliter (mg/dl) or your hemoglobin A1c is above 6, an OGTT is recommended. It is also recommended to get an OGTT if you have one of the following factors regardless of your fasting glucose and A1c scores: You score is 140 mg/dl or higher on a random glucose test (a non-fasting test), have a big belly, which can indicate a BMI, body mass index of 30 or higher, have head snapping slumps after heavy carbohydrate meals or have a family history of diabetes or heart disease.

A lipid panel is where you can begin to evaluate for cardiovascular abnormalities. A fasting lipid panel can look at your total cholesterol, LDL (bad cholesterol), HDL (good cholesterol) and triglycerides. Typical lab values dictate that your cholesterol should be under 200, HDL's between 45-50 mg/dl, LDL's below 130 mg/dl and your triglycerides under 150.

If you have a family history of cardiovascular disease or you have experienced some cardiovascular episode in the past, you would want these values monitored properly by your physician. I personally like to see LDL values under 100.

Inflammation is a silent killer and in Part IV I will go over how you can reduce inflammation with diet and supplements. To measure your inflammation level, C-reactive protein is a good test. Having inflamed arteries can lead to cardiovascular disease. Using a C-reactive protein test can indicate this if it is high. Since this test is very sensitive, if positive you should repeat it in about a month.

It's estimated that in 2008, some 180,000 American men were diagnosed with prostate cancer. It is recommended that men have their PSA checked annually once they hit 50. It is not a bad idea to have it checked earlier. I believe I first received the dreaded digit exam when I was 30. Since then I have had one every couple of years. If the doctor is experienced, it is not too bad.

Guys, don't forget your thyroid. Men can experience thyroid issues just as woman can. We live in a society where poor diet, stress and poor sleep patterns are the norm. This type of lifestyle will give your thyroid fits. You can have an overactive thyroid called hyperthyroidism. This can lead to an increased heart rate, anxiety, sleep problems, weight loss and a goiter (swollen area in the neck).

You can also have an underactive thyroid or hypothyroidism. This is characterized by personality changes, hair loss, weight gain and cloudy memory. The test to start with would be the TSH or thyroid –stimulating hormone test. Specific tests should be ordered for a more thorough evaluation like a free T3 and free T4.

Also it is so important to have your vitamin D level checked. Deficient vitamin D levels have been linked to problems with immunity, bone and heart health as well as some cancers. I will go into more detail in the supplement section later.

Ladies You're Up

Don't think for a minute I forgot about all you ladies that want to be healthy. Just like the guys, you need to get a comprehensive blood work up, checking sugar, lipids and thyroid levels. Also include vitamin D levels, a CBC, your body fat and blood pressure. Everyone should make it a habit to check their weight on a daily basis. It can make it more likely you will maintain a healthy weight. I like this strategy because I feel that you need to monitor progress or lack of it regularly. You always hear people saying that they do not want to get near a scale. What they are saying is that they either cheated or have given up on trying to achieve a healthy weight.

I also recommend that women take a daily multivitamin that contains iron and folic acid. A word about vitamins: they are not created equally. It is better to do your research and purchase high quality supplements. But higher prices don't always mean higher quality. I will go more into supplements later.

When you reach your 20s it is a good idea to see your ob-gyn for a breast and pelvic exam along with a Pap smear. When you hit the big 4-0, you should add an annual mammogram. If you are in your 20s, 30s or 40s you should have a complete physical exam every 2-3 years. For exact recommendation you can check with your doctor.

Understanding the Process

A word about the tests recommended and blood panels. The routines and tests that have just been presented are guidelines to allow men and women to reduce the risk of disease. My rule of thumb is to always work proactively with your health care provider on these strategies. Also remember they are preventive strategies of disease and do not represent wellness strategies. The difference between prevention and wellness cannot be stressed enough.

Regarding blood work, the lab ranges that you see on your blood report are usually determined by values of a large population of patients from that lab. Remember these might not be the healthiest of individuals. Lab values also can change from lab to lab and do not represent optimal healthy ranges. You need to have your blood results analyzed using functional ranges as well as lab ranges. Functional ranges are narrower values that can be used to see unhealthy patterns starting before they are pathological. And isn't that the name of the game?

HaleyHealth Action Steps Chapter 6

- Write down the terms "health," "fitness," "physical activity" and "exercise."

Now write down examples of each and visualize them. I like you to do both and really try to visualize examples of what these terms mean. What would you look like being healthy and fit? What is physical activity and what are good exercises for you?

- On a piece of paper make two columns. In one column, write down your fitness components; in the other, write the health tests that I recommend.

This should provide a nice basic blueprint for what your goals should be like.

Chapter 7

DO YOU HAVE WHAT IT TAKES?

Up until this point you have been presented facts and figures, recommendations, definitions and my own personal touch. You may be steamed, or pumped up and ready to go, but I have one question for you. Do you have what it takes? I love this statement. I love it when I heard it on the Armed Forces commercials and I love it when I hear it from a championship sports coach.

What does it mean to you reading this book? It means that if you reached this far, you really want to change your life. Change is a nice word and pumps people up. Whether it is said in elections or by team owners hiring a new coach, it just resonates. However, most changes are difficult. You hear people mention something is just a small change. Your boss might say that he or she is making some small changes around the office and not to worry. Well, changing your lifestyle from being unhealthy to the picture of health is HARD. Listen to me – it is real hard. But you know what? If you follow a good plan and increase your knowledge, I am confident you can do it. I am not asking you to split an atom, just get healthy.

Get Rid of That Victim Mentality

Before we get into how you can accomplish your goals I would like to bring up an old point. In a previous chapter we spoke of being a victim. In fact being a victim can result in a victim mentality. This can be a major obstacle in obtaining the health you deserve. In fact this type of self-sabotage can almost guarantee that you will never reach your goal. If for some reason you do accomplish your goal playing the victim role, it will be much harder.

A victim mentality can be defined as when a person blames everyone else for what happens in their world. It can also be defined as when a person feels that their future only holds bad things. We see this in health promotion all the time. It can be very subtle or it can be very obvious. In my experience, either way will block someone from being healthy. Let's look at a common situation that will expose this mentality.

The Subtle Approach

This example is a common subtle approach to this mentality that I see on a daily basis.

Mr. and Mrs. Smith come into the office with moderate back pain. I say moderate because I have learned over the years if someone is in severe pain, that is not the time to address their lifestyle. The first order of business is to try to lessen their current problem, and when they feel better we can address their lifestyle. The funny thing is they almost always say two things when they are in distress. The first is usually, "What is wrong with me." The second is usually, "I was feeling fine before the pain." In their life they think about symptoms or the absence of them as a measure of health. They are not trying to live to be healthy. Remember, crisis care versus health care.

In fact, as I write this chapter a patient came back in my office today. This patient has not been treated in several months. However, this patient has not been following up on his exercises and lifestyle changes.

Prior to today, he came into my office with severe low back and leg pain. He has degenerative lumbar discs with moderate herniation, muscle spasm and limited range of motion in the lumbar spine, hips and ankle. Additionally, he had limited neck and shoulder movement. You get the idea, he was one stiff dude. He also had a multitude of functional dysfunctions in alignment, muscle tone, balance and core weakness.

A specific program was designed to help him decrease his pain and increase his range of motion and function of the lower back. We concentrated on other spinal and extremity-related areas of imbalance.

Strengthening his core muscles to help protect against re-injury was also addressed.

This type of program was designed to first address the crisis (pain), and then help deal with the functional dysfunctions that caused the pain. The last piece of the plan was to address lifestyle, which would help the patient spare his spine and help him prosper on the road to wellness.

After a week and half of treatment when the pain was decreasing, and just around the point I was to introduce the core stabilization program I designed for him, he vanished. Only a few months later, he reappeared with the same problem that was never fixed properly in the first place. This patient failed to complete the recommended treatment plan, which I mentioned, was designed to take him beyond crisis and help him function better. When he returned, what two things do you think he said? "Why is this happening?" and "I was feeling fine so I felt I didn't need to come back." But you know what came back, "his unfixed problem."

I am not saying that if the patient's complaint is truly healed they need treatment, however they need to do their homework. Usually they feel that once they feel fine they do not need to do anything else. If your teeth feel fine right now, stop brushing your teeth for a while and see what happens.

This mentality goes back to Mr. Smith's case. The Mr. Smiths of the world come in with a series of underlying problems that require a more detailed answer than they want. They want to hear words like arthritis, sciatica, disc herniations, diabetes, colitis, etc. Even as bad as these ailments can be, Mr. Smith has heard them all before from parents, friends and relatives who have all been stricken in the past.

They can understand the condition terminology because this is how they were conditioned their whole life. They expect it to creep into their personal life at some point. Their logic is sweet, simple and right to the point. And you know it is something you just get. Aunt Betsy had lumbago, Uncle Charlie the gout and sister Sara is just not well.

The common denominator I see in this mentality is that it is not their fault. These are just things that everyone gets. Like getting sick as a child, it is not your fault. You go to the doctor and your condition is addressed in short terms and medication is prescribed. The conventional doctor rarely addresses the notion that part of the problem might be that all that sugar you're gulping down is weakening your immune system.

In Mr. Smith's case it's not the fact that he is overweight, overfed, underactive and a postural mess. No, he has disc problems and people get them. Like there are gremlins that just attack your spine.

The Less Subtle Approach

Most of the people I see that neglect their health will not do anything about it until it's too late. They do not want to change. They will get annoyed if you try to make them change. I have seen too many of this type. They are the true Impatient Nation, as they want someone else to do the work and do it now. They don't care about the future unless it is too late or an emergency. And even in that case, once the chaos clears they are back to their old ways. They are living crisis to crisis and are playing Russian roulette with their health.

Giving Up on Being Healthy

A perfect example of this is someone who has given up on trying to be healthy. That is your decision and you can live your life any way you want but understand the possible consequences. I once had an obese patient who presented with a host of health issues, least of importance was spine degeneration. However, I would spend time with him to discuss lifestyle changes only to have it fall on deaf ears. He would repeatedly present with the same problems, which lasted for many years.

He would get better, then worse, and then better again, until he became so bad he needed emergency medical treatment. When he came to my office a few days after his trip to the ER, he was distressed. He then asked me two questions I mentioned earlier, which showed he never listened. He asked, "How did this happen?" and "I was feeling fine for a while." He like many, did little to change his lifestyle and when he was desperate for answers I one last time tried to encourage him that he needed to change his lifestyle. He responded with, "I am not going to change," "I like to eat, and I don't like to exercise." To the sick care business this one is yours.

Defeat of the Victim Mentality

You can break out of a victim mentality. This is a must to succeed in improving your health. I don't want you to think all patients are negative and hopeless. That would be a disservice to all the fine people I have served and who have allowed me to assist them in improving their lives. Also, it would be a disservice to all the true health providers that make a difference. However, we still have a tough battle ahead. Don't play the victim role.

The victim mentality is hard to break but easy to notice. It seems some victims like the attention victimhood gives them. I have met many people that without listing their woes they would have nothing to say. I remember a patient once told me that when she attended a reunion everybody was talking about all their aches and pains. This attention seems to validate their existence.

You have to rise above being a victim. It is not acceptable playing the victim role when you can help yourself. An example is when I review recommendations to a patient and it goes in one ear and out the other. They continue to complain about their problem and not listen to any solutions.

Understand that in trying to change your mentality you can slip from time to time. Accept it and continue on with your mission. Remember: the strong shall survive.

Also remember that Winston Churchill said, "The price of greatness is responsibility." That statement sums it up.

Let's Accomplish Your Goals

Now that you have stripped down that victim mentality, let's accomplish your goals. In my opinion you really have to want it. And that is hard because there are so many distractions out there. You have to have a great support system in place to succeed easier. You can succeed on your own but it is much harder.

First you have to visualize yourself achieving the goal. See it first before it happens. This is a common technique used by athletes and many successful people. You can spend some time everyday visualizing yourself in a healthy state of mind and body. You can also use a poster board and cut out pictures of what you want to be. Or get books with healthy pictures to motivate you. I routinely have pictures, books and articles that I refer to for motivation.

Commit to achieving the goal by writing it down. Fail to plan; plan to fail. Read my lips, you have to do this and refer to this over and over until you succeed. Remember, it is not a real goal until it is written down.

Establish times for checking your progress in your calendar system. This is extremely important and reflects the responsibility I am looking for in you. You need to evaluate your progress regularly. Also you have to be able to handle any failures you might have along the way. If you don't accomplish your goals on time, you must remain calm, cool and collected. You need to figure out what went wrong and how to fix it. Setbacks happen; don't let them stop you. Just analyze the situation and move forward. Sometimes you have to take a few steps back before you go forward.

Reviewing your progress is also essential, like checking your weight everyday. I know some nutritional specialists disagree on this point. My reason is because people genuinely can get foolish and wimpy in certain situations. Case in point, when someone has cheated on their nutritional program, they are afraid to get on the scale. You hear this all the time. "I am so afraid to get on that scale."

That is a great strategy—just avoid the scale and all will be well. You have to become an expert on your lifestyle and how your body reacts. Daily weigh-ins let you know what you can and cannot do if you are to succeed. Maybe a little less at the cocktail hour you attend might help. These are the things you realize when you hit the scale regularly.

Tying Goals to Your Health

Now you can apply similar steps to achieve your health care goals. You can see that they are about changing your attitude and lifestyle. We are getting there. It is starting to come together so pay attention. Goal setting is goal setting no matter what the outcome is to be. You do not set goals to lose. Well maybe if you are a sports team looking for the number one pick in the draft, but for our purpose we win.

First you have to develop the desire to be healthy. You have to develop this desire down deep into your core. People with a deep

desire set difficult goals. I remember watching Michael Jordan playing a 1997 NBA finals game against the Utah Jazz. Jordan was very
sick with the flu, but he played anyway. The result was of course
another stellar Michael Jordan performance and a Chicago Bull victory. During the post game interview on the court, Jordan, who was
practically doubled over from exhaustion, was asked how he pulled
off such a great game while feeling so sick. He said, "I wanted it
really bad." That's desire.

With desire comes belief. You have to believe in yourself 100%, not
75% or 50%, but 100%. If you go half speed you will get half the result.
Believe in yourself and others will start to belief in you. It is like writing
this book. I am not an author. Writing to me is boring. I can talk up a
storm, but I have to put it down on paper for it to be real. The more I
mentioned to my friends and patients that I have a desire to write a book
the more they believed I meant business.

I mentioned writing it down makes it real. If you write your goals
down and reflect on what you wrote on a daily basis, they become real. I
looked at the outline of this book daily and visualized not only what the
finished product would look like, but also how it would feel. An outline
is basically a list of your plan to succeed. Make a roadmap for your goals
and how you are going to feel during the process. How are you going
to feel after you drop twenty pounds and have more energy to play with
your kids? Moms, how great are you going to look in your new clothes?
You think maybe your husband would want to take you out on the town?
It will transform and change your life.

Plotting Your Outline to Health

In your outline make sure your baselines or starting points are known.
Once you know your baselines like blood pressure, sugar level, weight,
body fat, fitness level, etc., you can start to plot how you are going to get to
the ideal values. Set reasonable deadlines to achieve these attainable short
term goals. If you have really high blood pressure or have a sugar problem,
you need some time to fix it. If you need to lose 100 pounds, give it time.
However, strive to reach your deadlines and understand how you did it.
Because once you succeed, you want to tell others and teach them.

Break Through Any Roadblocks

You also need to anticipate the possible roadblocks that could get in your way. It's rare that everything runs as smooth as planned. I was at a seminar once when the presenter was talking about proper nutrition and weight loss. He mentioned that he was spending a lot of time with his clients about dealing with obstacles. In this instance, it was late fall and the holidays were approaching, which is a common time people go off the nutritional deep end. But, with proper preparation, getting back on track can be easier.

An Educated Mind Has a Better Chance to Succeed

Having easy access to information and support increases your chances for success. I mentioned early on in this book that you could get a wealth of information on the internet, libraries, magazines and newspapers. The more educated you become on a subject, the more comfortable you will be. When you start a new job, usually there is someone who shows you the ropes about the business. It is not that they are smarter than you. They just have more time learning the business and at that point have more knowledge on the subject. As you work at the business, you become more knowledgeable and more comfortable. The same goes for learning how to be healthier. Easy does it. It will not make you a doctor even though you may think you can play one on TV. However, you will be more knowledgeable about your health than the average person.

Find Some Motivation

Most people I know, including myself, are more motivated when there's a certain event or reward to shoot for. It is not uncommon for someone to decide to get in shape for a wedding or a high school reunion. Many people get the fitness bug to participate in a sporting event like a race or to join a team. I had a patient quit smoking cold turkey once she had kids. Identifying your motivation is extremely important.

National Weight Control Registry

Another way to keep on track is to become a member of the National Weight Control Registry. I first noticed weight control registries when I came across a TV program featuring people who qualified for inclusion to a weight control registry program. It was very interesting because they were regular everyday people from all walks of life. However, they were far from typical. They succeeded in an area where many of us fail. They mastered the art of losing body weight and the ability to keep it off and get healthy.

One person featured had a whole closet filled with junk food but had developed the discipline to eat only a small amount, very infrequently. One or two cookies every so often as opposed to a whole box every other night.

The National Weight Control Registry is a database started by James Hill, Ph.D., from the University of Colorado Health Science Center and Rena Wing, Ph.D., from Brown Medical School. They set out to learn from people who had experienced long term weight maintenance. Remember, as we mentioned, this is the most important part. Many people struggle to lose weight only to have it regained.

The inclusion criteria for the registry is that a participant has to maintain a weight loss of 30 pounds for a least one year. Of the 4,000 participants, most were white women, 41 to 49 years old. Men comprised only 20% of the participants. Forty six percent of all participants were overweight by the age of 11, and a quarter, between 12 to 18 years old. This is more evidence about the importance of educating our youth about health. The data revealed that 28% became overweight during adulthood. Keep in mind that this data is for participants who lost weight and kept it off. As I mentioned previously in this book, the overall stats are much higher.

One important note is that 46% of participants had at least one over-weight parent; 27% had both. This shows the importance of a healthy household. Good habits start in the home. Like father like son, or more likely, like fatter like fatter.

The registry data teaches us many important lessons. The first lesson is that it is possible to maintain weight loss. The data showed that approximately half the people who lost 10% or more of their weight were able to maintain this loss for a least one year. And approximately 25% were able to maintain their weight loss for five or more years.

Lesson number two focuses on the point of making your goals realistic and sustainable. Most of the members of the registry modified their food intake so they could lose the appropriate amount of weight. The nutritional programs varied, but most people followed a diet that was reduced calorie and low fat.

The remaining lessons are similar to what has been presented prior. You have to exercise to lose and maintain weight. Members reported that they did the following: 94% increased their physical activity and exercise level; 76% walked as their main form of exercise; and 90% exercised for an hour a day. For these folks, maintaining weight loss was accomplished with calorie reduction and exercise.

Monitoring progress was also noted as being important, something that becomes easier as weight loss is maintained. Consistency was important too, as the data showed that members who ate consistently all year around and avoided holiday binges were more successful. After 2 to 5 years of maintaining weight loss, there is a higher chance it will be permanent.

Eating a regular breakfast was important. Half the participants were able to lose weight on their own, and half were able to use commercial programs for their weight losses. Finally, participants spent less than 10 hours in front of the boob tube each week, compared to a national average of 28 hours per week.

To help motivate you, I recommend that you have a tangible goal to achieve. Trying to qualify for the National Weight Control Registry is a great goal. You can enroll at www.nwcr.ws.

HaleyHealth Action Steps Chapter 7:

- Set your goals. By now you should be able to start to set your health goals – how you want to feel, how you want to look – and understand your health check numbers.
- Do all the steps mentioned. Go through the goal setting and victim mentality solution pointers in this chapter to set your mind right.
- See if you qualify for the national weight loss registry. Go for it, and see if you can be added to the registry.

PART III –
ATTITUDE
ADJUSTMENT

Chapter 8

ROADBLOCKS TO ALTERNATIVE CARE

"CAM" three letters you should be familiar with if you want to be healthy. CAM stands for Complementary and Alternative Medicine. Now what do these terms mean? Medicine sounds familiar but what does it mean when you preface it with the terms "complementary" or "alternative." This terminology can be difficult to define since it can have many broad aspects to it. The National Center for Complementary and Alternative Medicine (NCCAM) defines CAM as a group of diverse medical and health systems, practices and products that are not generally considered part of conventional medicine.

Conventional Medicine is Abundant in Crisis

Conventional medicine is usually called western or allopathic medicine. It usually includes MDs (medical doctors) and DOs (doctor of osteopathy). It also includes allied health professionals such as physical therapists, psychologists and registered nurses, among many others. These groups are technically considered more mainstream. They are abundant in a crisis care model.

Complementary and Alternative Forms of Care

The term complementary medicine practices refer more to, "being used along with conventional medical practices." In most of my observations, CAM treatments used by Americans are complementary. The term alternative medicine refers to the use of CAM in place of conventional medicine. The term integrative medicine is becoming popular especially on radio and TV shows. Just about every health related radio show I listen to in the car is sponsored by a medical professional that practices integrative medicine. This approach combines conventional and CAM treatments for the best result. In my experience it usually involves more nutritional therapy and less medication to deal with health issues.

CAM on the Rise

This trend seems to be on the rise as the numbers have grown over the past 10 years. In 1997 Americans made 627 million visits to CAM practitioners, as compared to 386 million visits to their family doc. They also spent $27 million out of pocket. These numbers have growth as compared to prior numbers looked at in 1990. The increase in the use of CAM from 1990 to 1997 was 47.3%. And we are continuing to see the numbers climb.

In a 2007 government survey, Americans spent $33.9 billion on complementary and alternative medicine over a 12 month period. The amazing point of this fact is that those dollars spent on CAM were out of pocket dollars. This meant that people thought so much of CAM treatments that they were willing to reach into their pocketbooks and spend, baby, spend. This amount was being amassed by approximately 38% of adults. This shows the willingness of Americans to look outside the box to help deal with their diseases and conditions.

Middle-aged adults appear to be most active in using complementary or alternative medicine. A study done at Wake Forest School of Medicine and the University of North Carolina at Greensboro looked at data from a CDC survey of 30,785 adults. The average age of the participants was 45, with an even distribution between men and woman. People were questioned on their use of any of 28 complementary or alternative therapies. The therapies were placed into six categories: alternative medical systems, biologically based therapies, body-based methods, mind-body interventions, energy therapies and self prayer.

The researchers found that the most frequently used therapies were self prayer, biologically based therapies, and mind-body interventions. They also found that middle-aged adults were using CAM methods more often than older Americans. There was an exception of self prayer that was commonly used by those adults that were 65 and older.

This proves one of my observations. Older individuals tend to resist change and stick to their old medical beliefs. However, I also feel that with the numbers improving and with people's acceptance of CAM, there is definite hope for future generations.

CAM for Crisis

Before I continue I want to make some important distinctions regarding the use of CAM. Remember the premise of this book is to reach optimum health for yourself and family. It is great that many people are using CAM treatments to deal with their ailments rather than relying solely on conventional means. In my opinion, CAM approaches should be added in battling your ailments. However, don't confuse this approach with a wellness approach.

If you use CAM to deal with health issues and do not address the underlying problem you are still engaging in a crisis care philosophy. Instead of treating your ailment with medicine you are trying a more natural approach. This is great, but it is like having a good offense but a lousy defense in sports. You are trying to improve your offensive attack on a problem (crisis), but your defense is weak and is allowing the problem to exist in the first place (poor immunity, resistance, etc.).

Let's look at an example that will help you understand this point. Suppose you have elevated blood pressure and high triglycerides due to your lifestyle. You have a couple of treatment options. You can take medication to reduce your numbers and mask the underlying problem, which is lifestyle. You can go on a nutritional regime that should include diet modification and there are also supplements that can help lower your numbers.

However, if you decide to go on a heavy supplement routine instead of medication but you don't change your diet and lifestyle, that may help lower the numbers, but it won't address the cause. Without addressing the cause, you really are not well. Once you stop the supplements, just like stopping medication, the problem can come back. It's that "pill for a problem" mentality, only using natural means like supplements as opposed to medication. This is a much better approach to try first, in my opinion. But go for the cause and you will be addressing a more wellness-based approach than a reactive one.

Five Categories of CAM

CAM can be broken up into five categories as classified by the NCCAM. These categories are: *Alternative Medical Systems, Mind-Body Interventions, Biologically Based Therapies, Manipulative and Body-Based Methods, Energy Therapies.* Some more details on these categories are as follows:

Alternative Medical Systems are described as complete systems of theory and practice. These alternative systems usually have evolved apart from the conventional American medical approaches and have origins in non-western cultures. Examples of these systems would include traditional Chinese medicine and Ayurveda.

Mind-Body Interventions are a variety of different techniques that are used to enhance the mind's ability to affect body function and symptoms. Some examples are: mediation, prayer, mental healing, art, music and dance that is used for therapeutic benefits.

Biologically Based Therapies use natural substances such as herbs, foods, vitamins and minerals. These therapies you should be familiar with, as they are found in most health food stores.

Manipulative and Body-Based Methods are techniques that are based on manipulation and/or movement of one or more body parts. This would include my specialty, chiropractic, also osteopathic manipulation and massage therapy. Also should be noted the various soft tissue techniques that are used by manual therapists like, massage, active release technique (A.R.T), neuromuscular reeducation, Nimmo, strain counter strain, proprioceptive neuromuscular facilitation (PNF), etc.

Energy Therapies use energy fields for healing purposes. There are two types: bio-field therapies and bio-electromagnetic-based therapies.

Bio-field therapy is intended to affect energy fields that surround and penetrate the body. These techniques can be done by applying pressure and/ or manipulating the body by placing the hands on or through these fields.

Bio-electromagnetic-based therapy uses the unconventional use of electromagnetic fields. This therapy uses pulsed fields, magnetic fields, and alternating current or direct-current fields.

A Closer Look at Some CAM Therapies

Looking at some of the popular CAM therapies, we can see certain differences from conventional medical care. Ayurvedic medicine has been practiced in India for the last 5,000 years. It is a system, which combines an equal emphasis on body, mind and spirit. It uses diet, exercise, yoga, meditation, herbs, massage and medication to help place a person in a state of harmony with their environment.

Three therapies that I feel are very interesting and beneficial, but in my opinion, not commonly understood by the general public are: traditional Chinese medicine, homeopathy and naturopathic medicine. I have very little knowledge and experience with traditional Chinese medicine, which has been practiced for over 3,000 years, and uses medicinal herbs, acupuncture and exercises like Qi Gong.

I have received acupuncture treatments and felt they were very beneficial. Patients often ask me if something like acupuncture will work. I say, work for what. They usually reply by naming their ailment, like headaches, sciatica, pain or whatever. Basically that is symptom (crisis) control, not wellness. My answer is the same with treatment plans or therapies I recommend. I say that people can respond favorably from various treatments. It depends on the individual situation, the skill of the provider and if the patient is a responder or not.

Whether it is CAM or Conventional, Nothing is 100%

We have to see if treatments that I suggest are appropriate and we have to see if you are a responder. If people are seeking some form of pain relief we can monitor that. To clarify my point, when a treatment is prescribed by a qualified professional it is usually appropriate to undergo a course of care. Then re-evaluations or follow-ups are done to check progress or lack of it. If everything prescribed, whether it is nutrition, medicine, chiropractic or any other established protocol, worked 100 percent of the time, follow-up exams would be irrelevant.

People respond different to situations. Health providers should instill a sense of confidence in their procedures, if appropriate, but going overboard is not proper in my opinion. Everyone can make a mistake even when trying to do the right thing. However, a doctor losing focus due to arrogance can lead to problems. So the moral of the story is that certain treatments can be of benefit. Everyone can respond differently to them. In my opinion, if the procedure is considered a lower risk you can make a decision with your provider. For the big risk stuff, like invasive surgery, get a second or third opinion to be safe.

Homeopathy and Naturopathic Medicine

I had some homeopathy treatments when I was in grad school, and I have great respect for this field, as I also do for naturopaths. I attended a nutritional seminar taught by a naturopath and it was one of the best seminars I have ever attended. Honestly, the knowledge that I experienced in lectures from "so called alternative providers or approaches" has been incredible.

Homeopathy was developed in the early 1800s by the German physician, Samuel Hahnemann. It is based on the treatment of the individual. It can be very effective on hay fever, digestive concerns, respiratory infections and other common maladies.

Naturopathic medicine has a strong belief in the body's inherent ability to heal itself. It seeks to find the causes of the disease rather than just suppressing the symptoms. This approach sounds extremely familiar with another very popular health system we will discuss later. Naturopaths use approaches such as diet modification, herbal medicine, homeopathy, acupuncture, hydrotherapy, massage and lifestyle modification to heal their patients.

Chiropractic – More Than Just For Sore Backs

Another extremely popular health care system is my main specialty, chiropractic. The American public heavily uses chiropractic, but we still have our skeptics. That is unfortunate because chiropractors provide a great service and patient satisfaction surveys are usually very high. If you are familiar with sports, most professional teams use a chiropractor to provide care to their athletes. And if we were not getting the results, we would have been out a long time ago. I have been fortunate to work on some of the world's top athletes over the years and have seen the benefit first hand.

Chiropractic was developed by Daniel David Palmer in 1895, ironically the same year the x-ray was developed. X-rays are one of the tools a chiropractor uses when necessary to assess the spine. After assessing the spine and/or related extremity joints the chiropractor performs chiropractic adjustments to help align and free up the affected joints. This will in turn help alleviate pain and help restore general health by reducing irritation to delicate spinal nerves.

Chiropractic principle is based on the premise that humans possess an innate healing potential and that disease can be dealt with by releasing this potential. Chiropractors look for the cause of a patient's problem as opposed to the effects. Sounds similar to many of the CAM practitioners we reviewed.

Working Together

You can see from these examples that there are many differences between modern traditional medical care and the alternatives. If health care providers of different disciplines work together, the patient will be the benefactor. This is a true complementary approach to health care. However, as I see it, we are not there yet and have a long way to go. Now we do have a lot of multidisciplinary centers opening up and medical doctors are starting to open up to the alternatives. This is a good thing.

The Wilk Case

Things in my profession have eased up slightly since we were at war with the medical profession. To give you a little history, you have to know about the Wilk case. When I was in chiropractic school this was the biggest case we ever heard about. It was a resounding victory for chiropractors and indirectly our fellow practitioners that did not fall under the conventional medical umbrella. The Wilk v. American Medical Association case was a federal antitrust suit brought against the AMA and 10 co-defendants by a chiropractor, Chester A. Wilk, DC.

Until 1983, the AMA position was that it was unethical for MDs to associate with what they claimed to be an "unscientific practitioner." And of course chiropractic was deemed unscientific. Before 1980, the AMA Principle 3 of medical ethics stated: "A physician should practice a method of healing founded on a scientific basis; and he should not voluntarily professionally associate with anyone who violates this principle."

While the Wilk's case was going on, in 1980, Principle 3 was revised to state that a physician "shall be free to choose whom to serve, with whom to associate, and the environment in which they provide medical services." Up until 1974, the AMA had a committee on quackery, which challenged what it considered to be unscientific forms of healing. One of the accused targets was chiropractic.

To go pass all the legal mumbo jumbo, after a decade of litigation and two court trials it was determined that the American Medical Association engaged in a lengthy, systematic and unlawful boycott designed to restrict cooperation between MDs and chiropractors. This was done to eliminate the profession of chiropractic.

I bring up this point to let you know there was a real battle going on. The medical profession was at war with chiropractic. It could have easily have been any other alternative health profession. Look how far we have come today. I was recently listening to the radio and a prominent insurance company was advertising that they cover chiropractic and acupuncture. There is hope.

Still Some Disconnect

However, I feel there is still a disconnection between conventional medical and CAM providers. At this point, I feel it is more of a lack of knowledge in CAM than a plot to eliminate a profession or two. In my own community, I can count of my hand how many referrals my office sees directly from medical doctors. This is despite the fact that I attained four college degrees, have been named a top provider in my field numerous times and have worked with the United States Olympic Sports Medicine program.

It is also difficult to get one of these providers to return phone calls on the care of mutual patients. It is frustrating when a patient asks me if

I've spoken to their doctor yet, and I've been waiting days for a call back. If I am lucky to get their doctor on the phone after constantly reaching out, their answer is usually they were busy. That might seem reasonable; however, when I recently went to specialist for a basic check-up, he took three calls from other doctors during my five-minute exam. If I do get a referral it is usually those cases that are sent as a last resort.

Physicians' Views on Complementary Medicine

With CAM becoming more popular over the years, physicians cannot duck the subject. The reason is results. These methods have been around as long as they have due to results. No matter how much someone tries to discredit CAM, it stays around because of results. In a survey published in 2002, 76% of physicians reported they have patients that use CAM. In that survey, 59% of them had patients ask about specific types of CAM therapies, and 48% actually offered a recommendation. Amazingly, 24% of physicians themselves have used some kind of CAM and said their own personal experiences prompted their recommendations. Just think of it: a quarter of medical doctors have used some sort of a CAM treatment.

Equally as amazing to me was the fact that 84% thought that they needed to learn more about CAM to be able to adequately address this topic with their patients. This is a tough subject because I think that from what I hear, there is not a lot of education in conventional medical schools about CAM or alternative means.

Is the Tunnel Beginning to Open?

There is definitely some light at the end of the tunnel. Most insurance covers some form of alternative care and even remedies that are not covered are usually within reason financially. There is an increasing number of physicians that are using alternative means in conjunction with their medical treatments. In looking at the University of Michigan's health system website there is a nice amount of information on complementary medicine and I know that Ohio State has a complementary healthcare center. GO BIG TEN.

Many organizations, like the American Academy of Anti-Aging Medicine (A4M) and the Institute of Functional Medicine, are advocating a lifestyle-based approach to health care. A4M is a multidisciplinary organization, which incorporates a variety of treatments to help slow down the aging process. They conduct educational programs throughout the globe and have many prominent and progressive physicians in their group. They also offer a variety of certification programs that are available to many health and wellness providers.

The Institute of Functional Medicine is another group trying to improve health care in this country. They also conduct many different educational and certification programs for health providers who want to advance their knowledge of functional medicine. They produced a white paper, entitled "21st Century Medicine A New Model for Medical Education and Practice." It is a wonderful piece of concise work, which helps set a blue print for a more integrated and wellness approach to true health care. It covers the strengths and weakness of modern traditional health care and how a change is needed.

Now we discussed different alternative methods to care. We even discussed some of the obstacles for medical doctors and CAM providers to fully work together. We even saw some examples of hope with CAM being integrated. But continue to remember the concept we are trying to develop. It is a wellness mentality opposed to a crisis mentality. It is great to use Chinese herbs for maladies prior to using prescription drugs. And using acupuncture or chiropractic when you hurt is better than gulping down pain killers. However, using natural means to control ailments is still crisis care. Even if it is more natural and beneficial, remember you still must get to the cause of your problem. Why are you getting sick all the time? Why do to you hurt? How can your body function better? Let's Get Well.

Haley Health Action Steps Chapter 8

- Pick 5 types of CAM therapies and look up the definition, treatment mode and national association.
- With this knowledge, research to see if any practitioners are local. Keep this list as your potential healthcare team.

Chapter 9

YOU KNOW IT'S BAD FOR YOU

We all do it, well most of us. We know that certain things are bad for us but we do them anyway. Now there are definitely certain degrees to our behavior. It can be something innocent like having some cake when we are trying to drop weight. It can elevate to something as dangerous as driving while drunk. See, we are not that stupid, but we still shoot ourselves in the foot, sometimes over and over again.

Some of the worst habits we engage in are no-brainers for neglecting your health. Smoking, poor diet and sitting too much. There cannot be anyone in the country that can think that smoking is good for you. The same goes for eating a diet heavy on fast food and junk food. I admit, when pressed for time I hit the drive through. But as we will see later, there are much better choices we can make. Sitting on your butt too long is terrible for your health and your spine. Sitting in a flexed position, like when you are at a computer, compresses your discs and can cause postural problems.

In my opinion, you should get a complete physical on a regular basis. Make sure the tests I mentioned previously are included. Usually physicals are done annually if you do not have any health issues. And even once you finish this book and get healthier you still need check-ups.

I had a patient that refused to go to the medical doctor for many years. Despite my recommendations and practically ordering her to get a full work up she became nasty. Long story short, she had a major problem with dizziness and chest pains. (Hello, red flags anyone?) She was rushed to the hospital for heart surgery. She had no clue how bad her heart was. She was lucky she survived.

My point is, this near-death experience could have been avoided if she had known what her body was doing all those years. Just because you avoid bad news does not protect you from it.

As I mentioned earlier, you need to get annual check-ups. At least you will know where you are physically. If you avoid this procedure you will decrease your chance for health. Realize I said get check-ups and evaluations, not jumping into the medical model looking for drugs and excuses. Doctors can perform tests and evaluations to allow you to know what your physiology is doing. If there is a problem you can make a decision with your health team on how to resolve it.

Athletes are always getting tested to see how their bodies are performing. This makes sense; any little deficiency in performance can be the difference between winning and losing. In our case any deficiency can mean the difference between health and illness.

Let's Try to Relax a Bit

Another thing we need to do is relax. I tell people to do this all the time. It is easier said than done. Nowadays we live in a pressure cooker, usually on a daily basis. That said, some form of relaxation is mandatory if you strive for health. I once had a patient that was extremely stressed all the time. She was extremely tight in the neck and shoulders and suffered from headaches. All she talked about was stressing over doing tasks for others. I suggested she try to think of herself, relax and let others fend for themselves.

Now the tasks for others were not anything serious or life and death. People were just taking advantage of her good nature. Well, she came back after a nice weekend and her muscles felt like butter. All of my treatments could not get this type of response. Her mood was great and I asked what she did to achieve this change. She said she just relaxed all weekend and babied herself. The change from her decreased stress level was astounding. But sadly old habits are hard to break. Within a few weeks she was back to her old stressful self, and what else was back? The muscle tension and headaches.

I Just Can't Figure This One Out

One of the bad habits I understand but can't figure out is smoking. I understand that for many it is extremely difficult to quit. I remember the old saying I heard when I was young that "smoking is the easiest habit to quit, I know I have done it a thousand times." It brought to reality how people desperately try to quit only to start back up. This happens in part because smoking is an addiction. Smoke tobacco contains nicotine, which is addictive. It is not uncommon to see someone go for a smoke when they are stressed or hungry. I also hear a lot of people say they are afraid to quit because they will gain weight.

Smoking is a hazard to your health and we all know this. More than 400,000 Americans each year die from smoke-related illness. That is almost a half million deaths from smoking per year. It greatly increases your chance to get lung cancers and many other cancers and diseases. And if you smoke, you not only harm yourself but the people around you due to secondhand smoke.

I spoke to a doctor who told me that secondhand smoke is more harmful than smoking due to its temperature. It is colder and more harmful to whoever breathes it in. I did not confirm this but it makes sense. I have never taken a puff from a cigarette in my life. However, I have inhaled an abundance of secondhand smoke from my dad. My dad smoked like a chimney and always around us. He stopped later in life for about 20 years but always suffered with his lungs. I always had mild chronic bronchitis, so maybe there is a connection.

Secondhand smoke from a parent increases their child's risk of middle ear infections, (which I had a lot of when I was young), coughs, wheezing and asthma. If both of the parents smoke, their kids are twice as likely to become a smoker than a kid who has two parents who don't smoke. I know a long time smoker who quit cold turkey once she was going to have children and never started again; it's been over 7 years. Bless her: she realized what was important.

With all we know about the hazards of smoking, why do we do it? What's more important, is why you need to quit. Once you quit, you will feel a difference right away. Your senses will improve. Your food will taste and smell better. You will cut your risk of cancer, heart disease, stroke, lung and respiratory problems. You will be healthier and have fewer complaints. If these reasons are not enough to make you quit, how about greed? You can save a lot of money. If you smoke a pack a day and the cost is 5 bucks per pack (and that's on the low side), if my math is correct, that would be a savings of over $1800 per year. Consider it a tax credit.

Take Me Out to the Old Ballgame

As I type this I am watching the American League Championship Series. This brings to mind how I enjoy going to the ballpark on a beautiful afternoon watching a game. The atmosphere and smell of the ballpark drives me to crave the good stuff, or should I say the bad stuff. Hot dogs with mustard, beer, pretzels and soft drinks are common fare at the old ballpark. I do not drink alcohol; I have not had a drink since 1989.

When I go to a game I might drink water but it usually does not go with all that tasty ballpark grub. I usually drink a soft drink, and I usually like it in those large souvenir cups. We now know that soft drinks like soda can increase your risk for diabetes and obesity. But did you know it could harm your kidneys? Cola soft drinks contain high levels of phosphoric acid, which can be associated with kidney and renal problems.

A National Institutes of Health study compared the dietary habits of healthy people and those with chronic kidney disease. Among their findings was that the consumption of two or more colas a day was associated with a twofold risk of developing chronic kidney disease.

Alcohol intake can cause brain damage, as well as a myriad of physical compromises. Now, I did not say alcohol abuse, because some impairment can be detected after only one or two drinks. These can resolve quickly once you stop. However, for those who drink heavily over a long period of time, problems can last long after they hop on the wagon.

If you have been around anyone that has had one too many drinks, you've seen the effects. Alcohol affects your brain, slurring speech, blurring vision, slowing reaction time and impairing memory, nothing you should be looking for if you want to be healthy.

There are many factors that can influence how one responds to alcohol, including the amount someone consumes, how often they drink, the age they started to drink, etc. Your state of health will also play a role in how your body responds, as will your age, gender, genetics and family history. We all go through days when we joke and say we are losing our minds, but excess alcohol will really do it.

Now, what about your poor liver? It is well known that alcohol abuse can trash your liver. And you need your liver. It is mostly responsible for breaking down the alcohol you consume and clearing it from the body into harmless byproducts. Excess alcohol can cause liver dysfunction, which can lead to diseases like cirrhosis of the liver and cancer. It is sad to see kids abusing alcohol, and increasing their risk of having problems.

Avoid Like the Plague

As I mentioned previously, one substance that can play havoc on your health is high fructose corn syrup (HFCS). There is some controversy brewing with this over abundant ingredient. I call it over abundant because it is found in most of the foods Americans eat. It is found in soda, fruit juices and most of the processed foods consumed. The controversy is real. The producers of HFCS have asked the FDA to change the name to corn sugar. Can this name change have a specific purpose? Can it be a way to trick consumers? Maybe or maybe not. Excess sugar is bad for you but we are hearing the claims that HFCS is worse. With manufacturers sensing this, can they be trying to head toward the lesser of two evils, as least in name?

It is also controversial because some claim that it is the same as table sugar. In fact, a 2008 report by the American Dietician Association concluded that HFCS syrup is "nutritionally equivalent to sucrose." However, there are many studies that demonstrate the health risk of HFCS. The consumption of HFCS has been linked to obesity, diabetes and metabolic syndrome. Two experts for further review in this area are Dr. Robert Lustig and Dr. Robert Johnson.

Fructose is a natural component in fruits and vegetables, but the fructose in these foods is mixed with dietary fiber, vitamins, minerals, enzymes and phytonutrients, which control the negative metabolic effects. What makes HFCS so dangerous is that it is consumed in huge qualities. This occurs because of the technological advances during the

1970s that made it cheap to produce. Since it is cheap to make it is put in many processed foods that are consumed.

Fructose does more harm to your health than sugar because of the way it is metabolized. First, HFCS is highly processed and contains fairly similar amounts of fructose and glucose. Fructose and glucose are metabolized differently in the body. Glucose gets metabolized by all your cells and is converted to blood glucose. Fructose on the other hand, is metabolized in your liver. When in your liver it gets quickly converted to fat and cholesterol. An over-abundance of fructose in the diet can cause fatty liver or even cirrhosis.

Sucrose or table sugar is a larger sugar molecule that is metabolized in your intestines as glucose and fructose. Fructose gets metabolized into fat in your body more rapidly than any other type of sugar. Most fats are formed in the liver. When sucrose enters into the liver it is stored, burned or turned into fat. Research shows that fructose gets turned directly into fat. This occurs by bypassing the process mentioned for sucrose metabolism.

What also happens is that the metabolic pathways that are used by fructose also generate uric acid. Fructose usually generates uric acid within minutes of ingestion. When uric acid increases over 5.5 mg per dl there is an increased risk for a multitude of health concerns. By now you can probably guess many of these problems. A good exercise would be to get a piece of paper and start to jot them down without looking. Then once you jot them down, see how many you get right.

First I will list the elevated uric acid problems then some others that can occur from high fructose consumption. The lists look similar, so let's go. Start to write and test your knowledge.

The uric acid problems include hypertension, kidney disease, insulin resistance, obesity, diabetes, fatty liver, high triglycerides, increased LDL (bad stuff), cardiovascular diseases, and pregnant woman can get pre-eclampsia. Also, elevated uric acid is found in gout.

Now here are the problems you could face from high fructose consumption. Metabolic syndrome, diabetes, high blood pressure, obesity, increased triglycerides and LDLs and of course liver disease, are all possible consequences of high fructose intake. Do you see anything strange about these two lists? They appear to be fairly identical to each other. They get you coming and going.

We talked about the fructose in fruits and the differences as compared to HFCS. But I like to eat fruit and isn't fruit healthy? Yes fruit is healthy and just about every suggestion on healthy eating urges you to eat more fruit and veggies. However, fruit contains fructose at different levels. Recommendations vary, but fructose intake should be limited to 15-25 grams per day.

That's not very much and you can reach that recommendation quickly. Some of the more popular higher fructose fruits are: dried figs at 23 grams per cup, raisins are 12.3 per half cup and seedless grapes at 16.2 per one cup. You can see just taking in these amounts will put you close to the edge.

I usually keep it simple with my patient's and recommend that they use a 3 to 1 ratio when consuming vegetables and fruits. That means for every three servings of vegetables you eat, you can consume one fruit serving. Basically it insures a much higher consumption of vegetables compared to fruit. It is also easier to remember and keep track of.

If you want more bang for your buck, here are some of the lower fructose delights. You can have a medium lime at zero grams. It goes nicely with some filtered water for a refreshing drink. If limes are not your bag, maybe lemons suit your taste. Indulge at 0.6 grams for a medium one. I like pineapple and I can make a wise choice by having a slice at 4 grams. So it is important to become familiar with what you are ingesting. If you were a racecar driver (I am a big NASCAR fan) you would want to know what is being put into your car. Try to do the same for your body.

Believe me it is hard but very doable. I just went to get some lunch and wanted something nice to drink. The place I went to had a huge drink section. As I looked at the choices I must have looked strange taking bottles out of the cooler and putting them back. Most of the stuff was loaded with sugar, HFCS or artificial sweeteners. With this poor reality it was water that won out. I was not too happy with the plastic bottle, as I will explain later, but you make the best of it.

Haley Health Action Steps Chapter 9:

- Make a list of any of the bad habits or foodstuff that you ingest.
- Write down the steps you are going to take to get it right.
- For one week, read every label available on the stuff you are consuming.

Chapter 10

DO YOU HAVE THE PATIENCE?

Patience is the state of endurance under difficult circumstances, which can mean persevering in the face of delay or provocation without acting on annoyance or anger in a negative way. Patience is a virtue and if you are going to embark on the road to health you need an abundance of patience. Being impatient, by definition, is not being patient. You are restless or short of temper, especially under irritation, delay or opposition. Being impatient as in the Impatient Nation, you will most likely fail. The reason being, that the journey from ill health and improper lifestyle, to being healthy is long with many twists and turns.

Bottom line it takes time to change and it takes time to heal. It takes time for your body to adapt. The time it will take depends on a lot of different factors. It will depend on your goals and current condition. If you are in relatively good shape and your health numbers are good, it should be easier to attain your goals. On the easier side, an individual may just need to eat a little healthier and drop a couple of pounds. This might not be a major production. It is harder if this same person decides he or she wants to complete in triathlons.

The time frame regarding health and fitness is an individual matter. The previous example could easily be reversed. The healthy and fit person that just wants a little edge might take forever if they are not motivated or if they are not comfortable with changing or adding something new to their lifestyle. And the person that wants to step it up and run a triathlon or marathon might be so motivated, that it becomes routine rather quickly.

It also depends on motivation, your current condition, resources, and how realistic you are. Highly motivated people tend to accomplish their goals more often than the unmotivated. I did not shake the world with that statement. However, when it comes to lifetime health and fitness, you have to be somewhat adaptable. If you are too rigid and too disciplined you might be miserable. Also you might quit if things don't go your way. I have seen people too gung ho, only to fail once they hit a roadblock.

Obviously, if you are in poor shape and really want to be your best it will be more of a project. Once again, no earth will be shaking on that statement. The more work you have to do, the more complex the task. You have to have a good support mechanism. If you have to change your nutrition and start an exercise program but don't have a clue it will be tough. You might need the help of a nutritionist or a personal trainer. But if you cannot afford these services it is harder. You can definitely achieve success with limited resources but it will require more effort on your part.

Don't Set Your Goals Too Low

Reasonable goals when it comes to your health are simple: Get healthy, period. Anything short of that is beneficial but should not be the goal. I see many people set their goals so low and it doesn't make sense. Now I am not saying you are going to be perfect and attain the ultimate prize. But go for the goal of being what you need to be optimally healthy. The health assessments we mentioned earlier, along with fitness ranges, should help you figure it out. Sometimes I hear people that are obese and do not exercise say just want to drop 10-15 pounds. Now a 10-15 pound drop would do wonders for them, but they would still be obese and inactive. That should not be the goal.

Set your goals too low and you can guarantee you will not reach any higher ones. When I was wrestling in college, my coach asked me what my goals were. After I told him I wanted to win the regionals and go to the nationals. He said your goals are too low. He told me to shoot higher and try to win the nationals. Unfortunately, it did not sink in and I only placed in the region and missed the nationals. I knew I was better than that, but set my goals too low and did not plan for anything higher.

Adaptability is the Key

In dealing with improving your fitness, here are some important concepts. Depending on what system you are trying to enhance, there are different adaptability mechanisms involved. I have to be honest; when it comes to fitness I am more of a weightlifter than an endurance guy. The important thing is that you do not want to be one-sided. Many people like to do just one or two activities. Believe me, I am thrilled when people take up an activity. Some like to walk in the park and others enjoy running. I will talk about exercise later, but I want to make a certain point now. That point is that to really be fit you have to work the components of fitness we talked about earlier.

To better realize this, take the example of me. I am big on the weight room. I was a competitive weightlifter and if I have my choice I would pump iron. But does that make me healthy or fit? No, it just makes me stronger; remember maximum strength. It also makes me more powerful and flexible. And it does wonders, when done correctly, on supporting my spine. However, it does not help my cardiovascular and respiratory system all that much. Now it can if done differently, but I strength train and do not work much on endurance.

When I was a wrestler, I was fit but unhealthy. Why was that? Well, with wrestling we worked all of the systems needed. We were in shape in regards to cardiovascular endurance, muscular endurance, flexibility, and even though we did not strength train during the season, we made up for it with our off season program. However, although we were extremely fit, most of us lacked real health. It was not uncommon to have many colds and sickness throughout a season. I had more ailments during my wrestling years than any other time in my life. The reasons were multifaceted. First, the extreme training that we did on a daily basis was brutal. We introduced tremendous physical and emotional stresses to our bodies. Couple this with extreme short term weight loss and contact with many other sick individuals and you trash your immune system.

It is important to be able to analyze your exercise program and incorporate all of the components of fitness into it. You walk around town and make great changes in body shape and health. But it may not help with much needed flexibility or strength. Likewise if you just work on strength and neglect your heart, you will likely run into problems. Also important is learning how to recover from exercise. In the example of myself while I was wrestling, I had very limited knowledge in recovery. I had poor nutritional habits, poor sleep patterns and did not utilize soft tissue therapy and massage work to help recover from the grueling training. Today we are much more versed in these areas. However, the average person does not use these techniques like they should.

Relating to fitness, your body will change and adapt according to the physical demands that you place on yourself. This adaptation takes time to see results. When someone embarks on a new fitness routine I usually say to expect to see noticeable changes in about 90 days. If you are a beginner that would be a reasonable time to begin to see your body change. But that is only the tip of the iceberg from a lifetime wellness point of view, so be patient.

Only the Strong Survive

To develop muscles that are functional and help maintain a good quality of life in my opinion resistance training is tops. Adaptive changes to resistance training are dynamic and will vary depending on the individual. To get the long-term benefit from resistance training you have to provide the proper stimulus to the neuromuscular skeletal system. The system has to be able to adapt and be fed further stimulus to improve.

A word of warning about weight training or any physical training for that matter. Your body could be sore in the beginning. Putting your body under different loads can cause soreness. The key is to start very slow and allow your body to adapt to the physical stress. Also you have to have good recovery skills. I always hear that professional athletes have all the treatments or modalities they need right at their fingertips, as compared to the average person. Well this is true, however, you also have access to the same care they get.

The problem is you have to pay for it. Well some services are covered by insurance. Pro athletes also seek services outside of the team locker room. More and more athletes are using nutritionists, personal trainers, acupuncturists, chiropractors, massage, etc. Plus many are using methods such as Pilates, yoga and meditation. So these services are not exclusive. They are offered to everyone, however they can be expensive. So if you do not have insurance or the budget for such services, you have to be more innovative.

Now getting back to muscle adaptation, how does your muscle change during training? First let's get into some basic muscle terminology. A muscle is broken down to smaller muscle fibers. Just like your clothing is broken down into individual fibers. When we increase the size of muscle and its fibers it is referred to as hypertrophy. The opposite would be atrophy. We have all seen atrophy if we ever had to wear a cast. Once the cast was removed the injured part was greatly reduced in size. As you began to exercise the muscle hopefully it grew back to the normal size. So in reality it hypertrophied in relationship to its atrophied state. To increase the size and strength more than normal is a goal of resistance training.

When you start a resistance training program you will most likely notice a nice little pumped up feeling in your muscles during your workout. This transient hypertrophy is short term and due to the accumulation of fluid and blood plasma. To start to develop some meaningful hypertrophy, you know some guns (AKA, Big Arms), it takes longer. It has been shown that to produce significant effects on your muscles it requires more than 16 workouts. On average most training session run usually 2-4 workouts per week with three times the most common. If you work out three times per week it will take you at least 5-6 weeks to see good results in muscle size. And this is just the tip of the iceberg. I tell my patients to dedicate at least three months, 90 days to make a significant change.

After they see the changes in muscle shape, they are sold. But you would be surprised how difficult it is for the average person to change their life and work on being healthy for 2-3 months. Many usually quit immediately or they hover. By hovering I mean they hop from routine to routine. They look for the perfect program only to keep failing because it is not the program, but them that is the problem. I like to say they hover because they might stay with a program just enough to get a feel of improvement, then they jump off. Instability is a sure road to disaster.

When you start to strength train the initial gains in strength are not a result of packing on muscle but from neural adaptation. You nervous system will start to adapt to your resistance training and kick in. Most people understand that their nervous system is important. However, most people do not experience such a dramatic stimulation of their nervous system. I explain to them that it is important to have a good functioning nervous system. And increases in strength are good for the ego. It lets them feel something is working for a change.

Muscle motor units consist of a single motor neuron and the muscle fibers that it innervates. Recruitment of motor units is the key to early gains in strength. This usually occurs in the 2 to 8 week range of early training. Long-term gains in strength are attributed to hypertrophy of your muscle fibers or muscle groups. Strength gains vary from individual to individual and may range from 7% to 45%. Remember this concept when setting your goals for training. Everyone is an individual and that means goals will be different.

Don't Forget About Your Heart and Lungs

Now we do not want to neglect your heart and lungs. You drive around your town or go to the park and what do you see. I see people running or jogging along. Some look like they compete in the many road races out there. I serve on the board of my local merchants committee, and we sponsor the annual "Lyndhurst 5K." I like it when I can get patients motivated to train and run in the race.

Most of us can run a little. It does not require a whole bunch of equipment, just good running shoes that you should check regularly for wear and tear.

You also should have someone trained in evaluating runners' mechanics check your running form. You can usually get a basic evaluation at your local runner's store like, New Balance or Road Runners

Sport stores. Most people do not have a proper walking pattern let alone a good running pattern so it's good to get it checked out.

Just like resistance training, getting fit with running or any other cardiovascular exercise takes time to adapt. The safe way to start is easy, and commit to staying with your routine at least two to three months.

The benefits of cardiovascular (aerobic) exercise are increased energy and stamina. It can help you control blood pressure, control lipids, and help burn those extra calories that you ingest. This is so important to maintain your ideal weight. I see many people trying to drop weight by dieting alone. This is so much harder and although I believe your nutrition is the most important element, exercise is a must. I always tell my patients that you have to combine good nutritional strategies along with proper exercise to hit your goal.

By increasing your cardiovascular capacity you will be able to work out harder. This is important, as I mentioned you need adaptation to succeed. Your body will become somewhat stale or steady if not provided additional stimulus. With aerobic activity you can increase the duration of your exercise to increase stimulus. You can also increase the intensity and frequency of workouts to increase the benefit. Activities beneficial in achieving this response are walking, running, jogging, swimming, rowing, gym aerobics and any activity that last long enough to gain an aerobic response.

Remember, just as with resistance training, it takes time to get fit. As you work out more and more, your body will adapt and you will get in better shape. Using a routine that combines some resistance training with cardiovascular work, you'll get more bang for your buck.

Controlling Stress is Crucial

You ever heard the term stress? Well of course you have. We are dealing with stress on a daily basis. I educate my patients on three major stressors that we come in contact with regularly. These stresses can play havoc on your health. I break it down to the most common stress elements: physical, emotional and chemical.

In further breaking these elements down we can look at what we expose ourselves to. Physical stressors are elements that stress you physically. Your occupation, workouts and postural positions are examples of physical stress.

Emotional stress is the one that we all know when we say we are stressed out. This is more of the mental stressors that we encounter. Examples of these stressors are worry, reaching deadlines, running a family, your job and emotional issues.

Chemical stressors are often over looked. Chemical stressors are elements that we put into our bodies either voluntary or not. Examples of chemical stress are drugs, whether prescription or recreational, poor nutrition, and environmental toxins.

The funny thing about stress is that there are good stressors and bad stressors. When you exercise properly your body is stressed in a good manner. If you take the same workout and become more intense than your body can respond to it can be bad. If your body cannot handle this stress it will respond poorly and break down. That means injury and overtraining syndrome.

How a body handles stress is best explained by Hans Selye's "General Adaptation Syndrome" or G.A.S. Selye was an endocrinologist who developed a three-stage model of the body's respond to stress back in the 50s. His G.A.S. principles have lasted to this day and while I was in chiropractic school we were schooled heavily on these principles. This is important because if your body cannot handle the stresses placed on it you cannot be healthy.

The first stage is the alarm stage. This occurs when your body responds initially to a stressor. This can be a physical, chemical or mental stress. The physiological changes to the body at this point can be faster heart rate, adrenaline rush, increase in blood pressure, heavy breathing, etc. In other words, your body jumps into action. We have all felt this when crossing a street and having a car head toward you. Or remember the feeling you get when taking a test you are not prepared for.

The next stage is the resistance stage. In this stage your body remains on heightened alert to deal with the stressor. The problem with this stage is that if the stressor is prolonged it can compromise your immune system. This leaves your body vulnerable to illness. An example of this is when you are chronically under stress or worry. Your body can feel run down. This starts to tie into the next stage.

The third and final stage is the exhaustion. During this stage your body tried to readjust to the stressors by releasing stress hormones. This tries to place the body in a state of homeostasis. Homeostasis as it refers to the human body is the ability to physiologically regulate your bodies' inner environment to ensure stability in response to fluctuations in the outside environment. If homeostasis is not achieved the end game would be a suppression of your immune system and possible trouble.

The title of this chapter asks you if you have the patience needed to succeed. I have presented information that shows you that to be healthy it takes some time. If you are not a patient person you are not alone. Why do you think the title of this book is, THE IMPATIENT NATION, there is a reason for it. So to help you become more patient here are some basic tips that might help.

- Get yourself a journal or organizer to write your tasks and appointments down so you can stay organized.
- Try to figure out why you are so much in a hurry. Examples are not getting up early enough, wasting time, need to chill out, etc.
- Pinpoint what are the triggers that cause you to be impatient. Also write them in your journal.
- When you get impatient, try to take a moment and relax. Most of the time it is no big deal.
- Try to remind yourself that things take time and unexpected situations are part of life.
- Take breaks from stressful situations till you are relaxed.
- Understand that with patience you have a better chance of getting what you want.

Accomplishing these steps can benefit you. The benefits from having patience are that reduction in stress levels makes you a happier and healthier person. You can make better results in your decision-making. Having patience helps develop better understanding and compassion. And having more patience can help you understand and appreciate the process of growth.

Congratulations. You have taken a huge step to being a more healthy and happy human being. I have presented you with facts, opinions and good old-fashioned horse sense to motivate you to achieving your goal. Now the fun part begins and it is time to work.

Haley Health Action Steps Chapter 10
- Read and re-read the steps for developing patience.
- Re-establish your timetable to achieve your short term and long term goals
- Get ready for part four and have fun

PART IV – THE HOME STRETCH

Chapter 11

PUTTING IT ALL TOGETHER

Congratulations, you have completed the first task in improving your health and changing your life. It is very difficult to try to change your beliefs and your lifestyle. I salute you for your effort.

With that in mind, I have made the preceding information fairly simple and straight forward. If you have to split atoms to understand it you will not do any of it. I have the average busy person in mind, so you can manage your time and dedicate a portion of it to your health. Even if you claim to be busy, remember, there is always some hospital bed waiting for you if you continue to neglect yourself. It is ironic how time will stay still if you are ill.

Change is tough and it will be especially hard on some. However, it is necessary and mandatory if you want to win. And if my words fail to inspire, maybe the words of a pro would help, ROCKY. In the movie "Rocky Balboa," there is scene in which Rocky is outside talking to his son. His son is having a difficult time living under Rocky's huge shadow, you know the blame game, excuse game, whatever, we have all been down that road. What follows is one of the most inspirational speeches to motivate someone to overcome their obstacles. You must see for yourself.

Crisis Care and Heath Care — There is a Difference

First, you need to understand the difference between crisis care and health care. This point has to be crystal clear. Taking care of illness, injury, trauma, etc. falls into the category of crisis care. This is usually handled by a crisis care specialist. Your teeth hurt, you go off to the dentist. Fall off your bike and break your leg, you are off to the ER, not the gym. You get my point. The U.S. has great providers and facilities for crisis care situations. But it is not to be confused with true health care. Trying to get your body to work and be at its optimal wellbeing.

If you are not functioning properly your health is diminished. It can vary in degree, mild stomach aches from time to time, occasional headaches, some back stiffness in the morning. We are to believe that this is normal. But symptoms are a sign something is not right. Still, we end up living with this stuff till we really breakdown. We can't eat without the antacids, we pop aspirin till the drug store is out. But that is considered normal if you don't understand health. By now you should, but if not let me give you a quick example.

Mary has Type 2 diabetes and has been on medication for years. That is crisis care and there is nothing wrong with it when you have a crisis. Providers are great for this, I like my doctors, but it is not health care. So one day Mary realizes that and starts to change the way she eats. She starts to exercise and reduce her stress. By changing her lifestyle, she helps her doctor reduce her medication. If she continues to improve, she might be able to get off her medication. That is going from crisis care to health care, real close to the ultimate goal: getting your health back.

You need to have a clear understanding that you are in charge of your health more than you think. You and only you will be able to determine that. The goals more specifically are to reduce your risk factors for disease, but more importantly be at or close to an optimal state of wellness.

You need to have an understanding on what health and wellness are. It is important to know that it is not only how you feel, but also how your body is functioning. Many people feel good but have a disease process going on. I see this all the time.

At this point, you must be crystal clear on you goals. They should be written down and reviewed. Spend time visualizing what these changes will do for you and your family. Will you have more energy to spend some quality time with your family? Is it the new wardrobe you have been looking at? Can it be just waking up without all those aches and pains? Or is it being able to work hard for your family? Don't overlook that one, because I see people scared to death about losing their job due to health issues.

Disability is no bargain. Whatever your fancy, a healthier life is the way to go. In this part, I will talk about some strategies that can help you get there. Most are from my personal experience as both a practitioner and a participant. Remember everyone is an individual and there is more than one way to accomplish something. I have tried to make it simple for you to incorporate into your life. The following components can be easily followed and are more for us average Joe's that want to live a superstar life.

Remember to also check with your physician before beginning any exercise or nutritional routine. Again, everyone is an individual and has different needs. Doctors should be excited that you are gearing up for some real health care. If they are proactive in health, they can even be a good coach.

How do You Conduct Yourself?

This is where we are going wrong. It all boils down to how we conduct our life. It takes dedication and focus. As I mentioned before, your mind has to be right. A great example of conflicting lifestyles was witnessed by yours truly recently. As I was stopped at a traffic light I happened to glance over at a sidewalk café. There was a family sitting at one of the tables eating their lunch. There was man and woman and a child. You remember, poppa bear, mommy bear and baby bear. Well, they were huge. And sadly, so was the child. They were hardly coming up for air. It was a long light.

As I was observing this, a dart shot by me. As I looked in my side mirror I could see a fit individual running down the road. (Remember the definitions of fitness and health.) As this occurred I looked back at the family still not coming up for air and I had one thought: lifestyle.

Now I realize we have all heard of people who have lived to a 100 and smoked, ate, drank and sat around their entire lives. Well this is true. Hey Jack Lalanne, one of the pioneers of American health and fitness lived to the rip age of 96. That is great news for the healthy lifestyle people. However, on the flip side, actor and comedian George Burns lived to 100. George Burns was notorious for smoking cigars. There definitely was a clear lifestyle difference between the two. Before you throw the book away claiming lifestyle is a joke, I have some important points to make.

- Yes, some people can get away with abusing themselves and others do everything right and have problems. However, they are the exception not the rule. Risk factors in lifestyle can lead to problems, which is why they are called risks. It is up to you if you want to take the risk or not.

- Quality of Life. You want to be able to have good quality in your life and not just longevity. Jack LaLanne was performing great feats of fitness and promoting health well into his advanced age. In a tribute to Jack, his lifestyle should be the standard we should strive for. I said strive for; a cheeseburger now and then will not kill you, but you get my point. Let's be more like Jack. By the way Jack LaLanne had a chiropractic degree.

- It really does not take that much work. Studies show that as little as 15 minutes of exercise a day can lower mortality rates.

What About Risk Factors?

Years ago I was asked to give a health lecture at my local high school. As I was going through my research, two risk factors, kept coming up in almost all of the diseases I was researching. These two factors were smoking and obesity. If we can just reduce these factors we can have a more Patient Nation.

I touched on smoking previously but it's worth more discussion. Long term tobacco use has been shown to cause a myriad of health issues. Among some of the more common are: heart and blood vessel problems, coronary artery diseases, heart attacks, strokes, lung disease and cancer. If you are pregnant and smoke some risk are: your baby can be born with a low birth rate, it can be born prematurely, have a cleft lip or you can have a miscarriage.

Tobacco is considered addictive due to its nicotine content. Tobacco also contains more than 19 cancer forming substances, mostly from its tar. It also contains more than 4,000 other chemicals. Really great stuff to put into your body, right? I hope you say no. Don't think that just because you don't smoke you are in the clear. Second hand smoke is in abundance if you hang around smokers. Inhaling someone else's smoke can increase your risk for heart and lung diseases. My dad smoked all the time and I never puffed a cigarette, however I think there is a connection to some breathing problems I had as a child. Also, my brother who never smoked had asthma.

Hey you want to go smokeless and chew. Well not so fast there cowboy. I am also a rodeo fan and seen plenty of chew. I tried chew once as a teenager and till this day cannot believe how sick I felt so quickly. Once was enough for me, but if you never learned your lesson here's what you can look forward to. Going smokeless can cause an increased risk of mouth and nasal cancer, gum and dental problems, as well as high blood pressure and angina.

There is a silver lining to your cloud of smoke. By quitting here are additional benefits you can hope to receive. Right away you should notice that your breath, clothes, hair, etc. will begin to smell better. This alone will make your world a better place; well a least the people close to you will appreciate it. Your senses should improve and the yellowness in your fingers and fingernails will lessen. Stained teeth will begin the slow process of becoming whiter. Hey you know what; your kids will become less likely to start lighting up themselves.

Here are some health benefits that should begin to occur once you put your last butt down. Your blood pressure and pulse should drop and the temperature of your hands and feet should increase toward normal. Blood carbon monoxide level should drop and your blood oxygen level should increase. Your risk of a sudden heart attack will begin to decrease. Nerve ending will begin to regenerate and your smell and taste should start to return to normal. As the months go on, your circulation will improve and you should be able to walk better.

As you continue to quit smoking your energy should improve, you should have less symptoms like, coughing, nasal congestion, fatigue and shortness of breath. After one year, your risk of heart attack is half of someone who is a tobacco user. As the years go on your risk of lung cancer and mouth cancer will diminish. And after approximately ten years, your risk for lung cancer death rate becomes similar to someone who never smoked.

Quitting is hard, but it can be done. The health benefits are worth it.

Control Your Stress and Improve Your World

If you entered a room of any size and asked is anyone stressed, you would see hands, feet and heads stand up. Why is that? Well, life can be difficult and hard to handle. It can keep coming and coming at you. If your body and mind cannot handle the load – PROBLEMS.

Most of the time, we stress out over nonsense. I have a saying, "don't sweat the small stuff". However, many people do and that will zap your health. If you always stress out over any little thing your body is always tuned up too high. And this is not a good thing. In keeping this simple, (I don't want anyone to stress out over this), we need to understand a little about stress response. Our bodies react to stressors differently and individuals can respond to the same stressors in different ways. In sports, certain athletes like Joe Montana and Michael Jordan seemed to be at their best during pressure filled moments. Others seem to wither away during these times. The common logic would be that they folded under the pressure.

Stressors will initiate a fight or flight response within your body. Your body will release hormones into the bloodstream, mainly epinephrine, or adrenaline and cortisol. Blood pressure and heart rate kick in and speed up. Initially in the short term this hormone response will make you sharper. It can boost your focus, memory and creativity. If you ever hear a loud noise while you were sound asleep you know what I mean. However, as stress continues a tolerated threshold is reached. Once you go beyond this threshold your body responses negatively and performance takes a hit. You might have felt this effect. If you undergone stress for a lengthy time you began to break down. The effects of stress on you can be abundant. They can include, but are certainly not limited to, a faster heartbeat, headaches, stiffness and pain in the neck and back, sweating, faster breaths and gastrointestinal and immune compromise.

Ways to help you manage stress are mandatory if you want ultimate health. I tell people you first need to eliminate, reduce or manage the stressor. An example would be if you have a bad situation like a job that you cannot stand you have to assess your situation. Can you get another job? Notice I did not say quit your job; that in most cases is stressful. It will also leave you neutral. You eliminated a negative but did not replace it with a positive like a new wonderful job. If you do not get that new wonderful job you are unemployed and will have other types of stressors. Remember, assess each situation. Maybe you cannot leave your job, so you might need to manage the situation better. Get more organized so there is less confusion. Get up earlier and beat that traffic that puts you in a bad mood to start the day with. Once again, assess the situation.

I love quiet time or "my time". After a tough day I like to drive and listen to the radio. This clears my mind and helps me sort out things. We need that 10-20 minutes of quiet selfish time. My office manager, Jen, once came to work at 5:30 a.m. to get her work done. She said it was fantastic to have her time without distractions. If being an early bird is not for you than you can spend your time by walking, doing yoga or breathing exercises or taking a drive like I do. But please pay attention to the road, if you don't that is one way to ruin your health.

Other important lifestyle changes that can help you manage your stress level would include: Try to get 7-9 hours of good quality sleep, eat a good well-balanced diet, and get enough exercise. Also try to avoid any negative expectations. Try to be positive and confident in your ability. Avoid the negative naysayers. The old saying that misery loves company does not work; you want to stay positive.

Focus on the Positive

Being negative or a pessimist can affect your overall health and well-being. But if you are on the negative side there is help for you. Some of the health benefits that can occur as a result of a more positive outlook include: a increased life span and lower depression rate, as well as, having better mental and physical well-being.

How can you reap these benefits? It starts with changing your thinking and attitude from negative to positive direction. First you have to identify if you are a negative soul. Many people think they are positive but are really walking on the negative side. Here are some forms of negative think or self- talk. You magnify the negative and filter out the positive. Is the glass half empty or half full? When the roof falls in do you blame yourself? Are you too hard on yourself? Stuff happens. Do you always assume the worst? Is that your style? Stuck in traffic and the whole day is shot. Are you trying to be too perfect? Is there no middle ground as you see it? Either it is good or bad or it's ugly. If you are not perfect you have failed. Ok so you are a little negative, so join the club. Here are some tips to tip the scale in a more positive direction:

- Hit the negative areas in your life and work on making them more positive. Tackle them one at a time.
- During the day do a self- check on your thoughts. If too negative try to refocus. Do this several times during the day if you need.
- Laughter is the best medicine, enough say.
- Surround yourself with positive people, AKA, winners. Positive thinking breaths positive thinking. Just like success breaths success and failure breaths failure.
- Don't say anything to yourself that is negative or lead to negative thoughts.

Nighty, Night

The next couple of topics in my estimation are under-rated for their importance in overall health. We need to get proper sleep as well as have to be able to digest our meals properly. Many of the people I consult with mention that they cannot get a good night of quality zzz's. And forget about their ability to digestion a meal without discomfort. We have talked about weight gain and obesity through- out this book and there appears to be a connection with sleeping patterns. In evaluating approximately 60, 000 women for 16 years during the Nurse's Health Study it was revealed that there is a link between sleep and weight. After 16 years, women who slept five hours or less per night had a 15 percent higher risk of being obese. This was compared to women who slept at least 7 hours per night. The shorter sleepers also had a 30 percent higher risk of gaining 30 pounds over the length of the study as compared to the seven hour sleepers.

There are other health problems that can arise from decreased sleep. In the short term you can experience a decrease in performance and alertness. Reducing sleep by a hour and a half in a night can reduce your alertness during the day by 32%. Your memory and cognition – how you think and process information can decrease. Stress levels can increase and your overall quality of life can suffer to name of few sleep deprivation problems. It is also estimated by the National Highway Traffic Safety Administration (NHTSA) that at least 10,000 auto crashes, 71,000 injuries and 1,550 fatalities can be contributed to drowsiness while driving.

In the long term, if you suffer from a sleep disorder, some of the problems you can face are high blood pressure, heart attack, stroke, obesity, as was mentioned and mental impairment to name a few. The good news is if you fix the problem and get quality sleep these issues can be reduced.

Some tips that you can do to help get a better night's sleep would include:

- Reduce noise levels and light while you sleep.
- Don't eat a large meal two to three hours before bedtime.
- Avoid caffeine for 4-6 hours prior to bed. Also, avoid drinking fluids before bed as this can cause frequency bedroom trips. If needed a cup of Chamomile tea is ok.
- Get regular exercise, but not before bedtime.
- Avoid afternoon naps.
- Calm your brain at least one hour prior to sleep by stopping to work on tasks.
- Don't deal with emotional or complicated issues at bedtime. Think about something relaxing.
- Have a well-ventilated and a comfortable temperature bedroom.
- Explore relaxation techniques.

There are some good natural supplements for improving sleep. I will comment on my supplement recommendations for general health later. I don't like to just give supplements for a problem without dealing with the cause. As mentioned before in this book, if you don't address the underlying issues, it is just crisis care in a more natural way, but it is still crisis care. That said, Chamomile tea is often used for sleep. My mother would give this to me at night and it was helpful. Melatonin helps with the sleep – wake (circadian cycles) to improve your sleep and valerian root is used for anti-anxiety and sedation. There are some reputable companies that have good formulations. However, as a disclaimer, you should always check with a qualified health provider and/or your pharmacist before you take supplements. They can help with doses, interactions and length of application. The local check out girl at the supermarket trying to supplement her income with supplement sales is probably not an expert. Just a thought.

Chapter 12

A PUNCH TO THE GUT

Excessive gas and bloating, constipation and stomach pains are not a pleasant experience. Nor are these ailments and many others normal. However, we consider them no big deal. How many people you know complain of some type of GI problem? They usually pass it off as not a big deal. Constipation, diarrhea, irritable bowel, etc. are prevalent and endured. Pass the antacids. If we have a problem we feel should get checked, it usually gets masked with medicine. We rarely address the underlying problem. This follows into the next area I will discuss, nutrition. I will review how you can reduce the inflammation in your body naturally with nutrition, as well as address the acid-alkaline balance we deal with. If you can understand and incorporate these two concepts, your digestion should improve.

Depending on whose information, you read 50-80 percent of your immunity lies in your gastrointestinal system. What we eat plays a huge role in optimizing this system and improving health. Our digestive tract, also called the alimentary canal, is a tube system of organs that runs approximately 30 feet (9 meters) in length which runs from the mouth to the anus, which includes the esophagus, stomach and intestines. It is responsible for digestion along with the liver and pancreas. This system is also responsible for delivering the components of the food we ingest to our body. Every piece of food that we ingest has to be broken down. It is broken into nutrients that the body can absorb and use. This process can take several hours for your food to fully be digested. Proteins are broken down to single amino acids. Carbohydrates are reduced to simple sugars and fats into fatty acids and glycerol. The water content of the foods we eat and drink get absorbed into the bloodstream for our fluid needs.

Poor diet, lack of exercise, medications and stress are among the reasons why digestion could become comprised. Digestive enzymes can be reduced and can limit proper food breakdown. Good or friendly bacteria located in the lower GI tract can also decline being in a short sided battle against pathogens that invade the gut. To help combat a failing digestive system, here are important keys that may be of help:

- Chew your food thoroughly.
- Take digestive enzymes and probiotics. I take digestive enzymes before meals and probiotics in the morning.
- Stay properly hydrated (if active try to work up to drinking water at the amount of half your bodyweight in ounces).
- Undergo a cleanse and detoxification protocol 2-4 times per year.

If you have persistent and more complicated issues an advance workup might be in order. I like to gather any medical records, lab work and detailed questions to develop a comprehensive program of nutrition and supplements to try to improve these issues.

The Power of Food

Boy what a true statement. We cannot overemphasize the power of food. Without the proper nutrients and food intake you will not survive. Ask those who ever went on a hungry strike how they did. Also of importance is how each food provides a certain response to the body. The timing of feedings and the circumstances in which we eat them is also important. People can eat a food like peanuts for example and feel fine. Give the same food to a person that is allergic and problems occur. You need to eat a certain amount of food to have enough energy to function, but overindulge and you can become an obesity statistic.

Knowing the importance of food is not a new concept. We get a little education in school as youngsters; however, in this country we have a problem. We love to eat. I am not saying anything shocking with this statement. It is ingrained in our culture. We get married, food, we die, others wait a little then after the funeral service they eat. Go to a football game and the best part is the tailgating. If we go to a restaurant and they do not give us enough to eat we don't go back. And other eateries brag about their portions. This atmosphere poses a problem. Real simple, overeating and lack of physical exercise is not the way to go. But you now know that after reading the "IMPATIENT NATION" and want to change. So where do you turn.

There is so much nutritional information out there it is sometimes confusing and overwhelming. Everyone from your next-door neighbor to your insurance salesman is a nutritional expert. It is the "wild wild west" out there and guiding yourself through it can be tricky. In this section I will cover a few of important principles that you can follow and succeed with. I strongly recommend that you seek evaluation from a professional expert in this field if you have any medical conditions I find it beneficial to have a detailed health history, blood work and any specific testing (e.g. Hormone, GI panels, etc.) so a more complete assessment can be make. At that point, specific nutrition and supplement recommendations can be made.

Nutritional Principle #1 – *Reduce Inflammation* - The first and major principle I recommend is to reduce the inflammation in our body with nutrition. Inflammation is a way that your body can fend off bacteria, viruses and other invaders intent on doing you harm. It also helps in the repair process of injured body parts. If you sprain your ankle it usually will swell up and hurt. It is basically inflamed. However, if inflammation is not properly controlled it can lead to problems. That is why if someone gets injured we try to control the inflammatory process with modalities such as ice, physical therapeutics, proteolytic enzymes, etc.

What if you don't perceive any real bad pain or have any noticeable swelling in your joints and tissues. Would this indicate that inflammation is not a factor in your case? Well let's investigate a little bit closer if I may. How's your diet? Do any of these relate to you?

- Are you regularly eating grains, grain products, refined sugar products and drinks?
- Do you regularly eat partially hydrogenated oils, cheese, daily and soy?

- Have a little too much fat around your waist?
- Tire easily, don't exercise regularly, get sick often and starting to look old?
- And of course, do you have any body aches, pain or soreness?

If you answered yes to any of these points — relax most people do — this also can indicate that your body is too inflamed. You can be suffering from a more chronic inflammation pattern that can be silent in nature until a symptom or crisis occurs. Chronic inflammation throughout your body systems can cause devastating degenerative effects. Chronic inflammation has been linked to many common illness including cancer, atherosclerosis, heart disease, obesity, diabetes, digestive disorders and Alzheimers to name a few.

The good news is that by controlling your diet you can help improve this situation. By reducing the foods that promote inflammation and concentrate on the foods that reduce inflammation you can change your inflammatory profile. The way I like to accomplish this is by using the information put together as "The Nutrition Foundation" guidelines. These guidelines and protocol are presented nicely and simply by Anabolic Laboratories (www. anaboliclabs.com) and Dr. David Seaman, (www.deflame.com).

Anabolic Laboratories is a nutritional supplement and education company based in California and Colorado Springs, Colorado, which supplies health care providers with high quality nutritional supplements. This is important because as healthcare providers we are dealing in a clinical setting. In that environment we can see if the nutrients and nutritional advice we give our patients are of benefit. This is a major difference from getting nutrients from off the shelve supplements.

We are walking, talking inflammation factories. The majority of the typical American diet makes us very "Pro – Inflammatory." That is not a good place to be as we noted some of the consequences with inflammation. Diet and your nutrition protocol will have a lot to do with changing this situation. The goal is to become more anti-inflammatory and we can start with some good solid nutritional concepts. Let me ask you a question knowing what we just covered. Would you want to inflame your body or defame it? I hope we all would like to defame ourselves so we can reach a healthy state. The amount of defaming you will need to do depends on your situation. The ideal approach and what is recommended would be to follow the guidelines to the letter and totally try to defame yourself. This is your best chance to become more anti-inflammatory and healthy. However, I understand that strict guideline beg for some cheating. Also, I know if you cheat too much you will just forget it. That said before I go over the basic guidelines on what foods to eat and what to avoid let me make my recommendations.

- If you have persistent body aches, pains, stiffness or soreness you need to de-flame strictly.
- If you have a health condition that can be related to chronic inflammation like hypertension, diabetes, arthritis, heart disease, metabolic syndrome, digestive problems, etc you need to de-flame strictly.
- If you are overweight or over fat you need to de-flame strictly.

Also make sure you are evaluated by your physician to see if the dietary changes are appropriate and make sure your condition is monitored. This should be done prior to changing your nutrition and monitored with your physician or qualified health provider. Once your current situation is under control you can loosen up a little. But remember if you return to your old ways your old self will appear. So understand the guidelines and live close to them if you want to maintain your health. Foods that are consisted pro-inflammatory or "inflaming" to the body should be avoided or significantly reduced if you have the signs and symptoms of chronic inflammation mentioned earlier. Here are some foods that have pro-inflammatory properties and should be avoided or greatly reduced:

Inflammatory Foods to Avoid or Greatly Reduce:

- Grains and grain products. Included are white bread, whole wheat bread, pasta, cereal, and any products made from grains or flours with grains.
- Partially hydrogenated oils. Found in margarine, deep fried dishes and most packaged goods.
- The following oils: corn, cottonseed, soybean, safflower, and sunflower. Foods that are made from these oils such as margarine, salad dressings, mayonnaise, tartar sauce, and packaged goods.

- Avoid sodas, soy, sugar and dairy. Use only in condiment size if you need to.
- Avoid meat and eggs from grain fed animals. Ok if meat and eggs are from grass fed animals. If you cannot get grass fed then use lean meat, skinless chicken, omega 3 eggs and fish.

I recommend that these foods should be eliminated from the diet for about 4-6 weeks, maybe more if you are very inflamed. After that period you can monitor your symptoms, energy level and overall well being as compared to before the anti-inflammatory protocol. As you become less inflamed and feel better you will have a clear understanding of how nutrition can affect your health.

You might be saying why do grains inflame? I thought whole grain products are healthy. Historically, our bodies are genetically designed to eat a diet consuming of fruits, vegetables, nuts, meat fish and fowl. You did not see too many bakeries in the cave man days or pizzerias for that matter. As we evolved we began to eat more grains. And as it became easier to process and package foods, we now have the product's that we have today and poor health.

Grains can cause a host of problems that have been mentioned when we discussed chronic inflammation. Some of the culprits are gluten, lectins, phytates. Increased inflammation, acidity and poor blood sugar regulations can be the benefactors of consuming too much grains. Gluten is a hot topic the last few years and with good reason. Gluten is a protein which is found in certain grains like, wheat, rye, barley and a host of other grain products. Gluten can affect people differently. Some people that are sensitive to the ingestion of gluten may not show any symptoms. Some might have only mild problems and others may suffer from a host of inflammatory conditions we mentioned before. While others might be suffering from "Celiac disease." Celiac disease is a genetic disorder in which gluten must be eliminated from the diet.

According to the Neilson Company, sales of gluten-free products increased 16 percent in 2010. Dr. Daniel Leffler, MD, of Harvard Medical School, estimated that approximately half of the 60 million Americans that suffer from irritable bowel syndrome (IBS) are probably sensitive to gluten. This is a critical part of the elimination detoxification programs

I conduct with my patients. The programs last around 3-4 weeks and patients must refrain from eating gluten, amongst other possible allergens. They also change their nutrition and take the proper supplements. It is amazing how well the majority of them feel. Then we can gradual allow certain foods back into the diet and monitor their response. This type of program gives you volumes of information on how your diet is affecting your health. It also identifies certain patients that still have health issues that may require advance work-up. My advice: while reducing your inflammation, bag the grains for a while.

Is There Any Thing We Can Eat?

By now you must be asking yourself: is there anything left to eat? Well of course there is. I would not let you starve to death. In fact, there are a variety of different foods to eat. I also understand that if rules get too strict they are more opt to be broken. So let us understand something. The prior list is composed of foods that will cause a pro- inflammatory response to your body in general. The preceding foods will provide an anti-inflammatory effect. So in essence you are either inflaming or de-flaming yourself as you ingest certain types of foods. Depending on how healthy you want to be will determine your willingness to cheat. If you are in good shape and have a good wellness and fitness profile I will not yell at you if you like a bagel or pasta from time to time. However, if you have issues and hopefully you honestly assessed yourself, then be strict till you improve. Once you are healthy, keep yourself in the healthy zone with improved eating habits. With that little pep talk out of the way here is a list of foods you can enjoy.

These are the anti-inflammatory guidelines I have been presenting to my patients for years.

Foods That Help Reduce Inflammation:
- All fruits and vegetables
- Fresh or frozen fish. I would avoid or ate sparingly farmed-raised tilapia, catfish and bronzini, which might have unacceptable omega-6 to omega-3 ratios and be pro-inflammatory.
- Meat, chicken, and eggs from grass-fed animals.

- Omega 3 eggs. Egg whites in general are also a good choice.
- Nuts: raw almonds, walnuts, hazelnuts, cashews, and macadamia nuts, etc. Enjoy, but go easy due to the calories.
- Spices like ginger, turmeric, fennel, red chili pepper, garlic, dill, oregano, coriander, basil, rosemary, and kelp, etc.
- Oils and fats: It is best to use organic oils. Use organic extra virgin olive oil and coconut oil. Butter is also a healthy choice as far as inflammation but I still use only as a condiment.
- Salad dressing: extra virgin olive oil, balsamic vinegar, lemon juice, mustard, and spices as mentioned.
- Whenever you are thirsty, drink water or organic green tea

A more detailed list can be found at deflame.com or anaboliclabs.com

I would like to give just a word of warning before you proceed. This is not to be used in the typical low carb mentality in which grains are reduced and protein is king. Look at the types of proteins allowed; they are anti-inflammatory. I have seen many people, including myself and family members go on the typical low carb diets. The mentality was, skip the toast but bring on the bacon, eggs, steak, butter, whatever. This type of eating mostly inflammatory proteins and foods can increase your inflammation and be counterproductive to being healthy. The guidelines presented help you reduce the inflammatory foods and eat the anti-inflammatory ones. This will help you achieve better vitamin and mineral quality, fiber content and quality protein for a healthier being.

Cool Breezes
<u>Nutritional Principle #2</u> – *Acid – Alkaline Balance*

As we continue with our nutritional principles it is important to understand the importance of balancing acid and alkaline. We all saw the harshness of excessive acid and what it can do. Remember the movie scenes where the good guy or gal was cornered by the villain and was able to escape by throwing some kind of acid in their face. Well battery acid may not be the best example. How about when I was a kid we would put a rusty nail in a glass of soda and watch it clean the rust off. That's a better example. And powerful stuff acid can be indeed. However, for proper digestive and body functions we need acid. The key is not to let it run amuck. If you have an imbalance of your acid and alkaline levels, which can be in the form of acidosis or alkalosis, depending on which level is dominant, problems can occur. The symptoms can occur as mild or non-existing or be more severe. You can experience nausea, vomiting, fatigue and breathing problems. It can even lead to seizures and even dead. If you are too acidic it can also affect your bone health, loss of lean muscle mass and increase the risk of osteoporosis. With alkalosis you can suffer from weakness, cramping and become irritable.

The measurement for this balancing act is called your "pH" level. The proper pH level should be 7.35 to 7.45. This is to assist that adequate oxygen reaches your body tissues. If your pH is below 7.35 you are becoming more acidic and if above 7.45 you are becoming more alkaline. The two main regulators of your pH are your lungs and kidneys. Also your intestines and liver help regulate your pH level in your cells and blood. Everyone should know their pH level. Your doctor can check this with lab work. You can buy home pH saliva strips and test yourself daily. Make sure it is a quality kit and follow the instructions to the letter. If not you can get a false reading.

The good news is that diet can affect your pH for the better or worst. The eating patterns that we already discussed will help balance your pH. By eating more fruits and vegetables and reducing grains you should have a good acid-alkaline balance. Just be careful with the meats and fish, as they are acidic. So if you have a low pH and are acidic watch to see if you are eating more meats than fruits and vegetables. I recommend a 3-1 ratio with vegetables to fruit throughout the day. So if you are eating two pieces of fruit I would like to see you have six veggie servings that day. Couple this with a small amount of protein per meal and you should be fine.

Does anyone object to this Couple Getting Married?
Nutritional Principle # 3 – *Food Combining*

When I was at a wedding as a kid, the priest would always say "does anyone object to this marriage" or something like that. I used to look around to see if someone had the nerve to say something. You know like, "he's a bum or she is no good." However, unfortunately for my childish entertainment I never heard those words. Maybe people are better off together than some foods.

As we talk about digestion, different enzymes work for different types of foods. When you eat foods in certain combinations it can disrupt these digestive enzymes and therefore disrupt proper digestion. One of the ways to correct this is to use proper food combining. I know it is not always possible to do this 100 percent of the time but trying real hard will really help you out.

This topic can get complicated so I will simplify it with some keys points you need to focus on:

- Don't combine your protein with starchy carbohydrates (breads, cereal, potatoes). If you follow the anti-inflammatory eating guidelines this should not be a problem, as we eliminated most of them.
- Protein and veggies are ok to eat together.
- So are vegetable and some starches like potatoes, wheat, rice, etc., but I would limit the inflammatory starches while de-flaming, as we discussed earlier.
- Fruits are to be eaten alone. I don't mean by yourself in a room or something, just don't combine them with the other food groups.

Do your best and continue to work these basic guidelines and you will *see the benefits*.

Don't Just Water Your Plants
<u>Nutritional Principle # 4</u> – *Water Intake*

It amazes me how little water people drink. This is even true with athletes. Your body is made up of approximately 60-70% water. When I was in school we were taught that you are approximately 72% water. That's a lot of water, and you need it to survive and function properly. Every year I talk to high school athletes about the proper amount of water they should consume daily. It is not uncommon for an athlete to lose 5-10 pounds of mainly fluid weight after a workout. I know this personally from my high school and college wrestling days. I know how much an athlete can lose from restricting their fluids and working out intensely.

The most weight that I lost quickly for a wrestling match was eight pounds in a night at age 13 and 15 pounds in two and a half days at age 16.

The most lost to make a certain weight class for a season was dropping from 170 pounds to 134 pounds in a little over a month at age 17. This is unhealthy and was predominately water weight lose not adipose (fat) tissue. My experiences do not even scratch the surface on other athletes weight loss episodes, but any way it is sliced it is unhealthy. To their credit, new weight loss rules seem to be in place now for high school and college wrestling.

These should help this problem significantly. I tell athletes to generally consume approximately half their body weight in ounces. So if you are 200 pounds and work out hard try to drink 100 ounces. If you are not used to drinking that much you can titrate or work up to that level. I also tell them to dilute it with some electrolyte replacement drink during workouts. A solution of 6% carbohydrate-electrolyte solution to water should be fine. This helps with electrolyte balance and can reduce dehydration and cramping. This is for athletes that lose a lot of fluid through their sweat. For an average person I rather you drink plain water instead of other drinks. If you have a filtration system at home that would be best. Also try to use glass containers instead of plastic if you can. The plastic leaks into the water and can be harmful. The proper amount of water would be around 3 liters or 13 cups for a man and 2.2 liters or 9 cups for a woman.

This varies depending on your activity level and health, but it is a good recommendation. The bottom line is to be hydrated and the best way that I check is through my urine color. If your urine is light yellow you should be fine. If it is too dark you could be dehydrating. There are plenty of urine charts that demonstrate the proper color. Also it you are taken medications or supplements your color could appear abnormal, so take note. One quick point is don't wait till you are thirsty to drink. By that time you feel thirst you have already began to have some fluid loss.

Too Much Of a Good Thing
<u>Nutritional Principle # 5</u> – *Calorie Restriction*

We love to eat, in fact we over eat. Unfortunately too much of a good thing can be harmful. Even if the foods you eat are the healthiest, if you eat too many calories and do not burn them up you will get fat. Oranges and bananas are healthy, but eat an excessive amount without burning the calories and you get fat. A study from the University of Wisconsin published in the journal, Science in 2009 showed that a 30 percent reduction in calories over a 20 year period was beneficial in slowing down the aging of rhesus monkeys. Now I know you do not want to wait 20 years and you are not a rhesus monkey but the take home message is reduce your calories, capice.

Well that is quite a nutritional blueprint. First you have a good list of foods to avoid and what to eat to reduce inflammation. Next you are set with your PH if you stick to the eating plan. You have learned how to combine your foods to aid digestion. Now you know how much water you need to be healthy. A quick point: some experts say not to drink too much with your meals as it will dilute your digestive enzymes. I find this is helpful.

Chapter 13

DO I NEED SUPPLEMENTS?

THE ANSWER IS YES!

This is a common question I frequently hear. Do I need to take supplements? The short answer is, yes. But understand what the word is supposed to mean. They are supplements and are meant to supplement a proper and healthy diet, period. Poor diet, poor supplement response. I know because I've been down that road. A few years ago I was the typical all-American: overworked, under-exercised, overweight, tired, sluggish, with brain fog, high blood pressure, etc. The funny thing was, because I have broad shoulders and some muscle tone, everyone thought I was in shape.

Well I visited a top-notch integrated medical doctor to get an evaluation. Prior to my appointment I received a packet of paperwork to fill out. It was comprised of a complete health questionnaire, diet diary, exercise history, etc. It was very thorough and I felt more wellness and lifestyle oriented than a traditional medical questionnaire. As I went in for my evaluation, the lifestyle part of the paperwork was kind of glossed over by the doctor. I was basically being evaluated in the standard traditional medical approach. This was fine with me at the moment because we all should know if we are healthy or diseased. Remember crisis versus health.

It was a good medical exam with a lot of testing, EKG, blood work, etc. After the exam the doctor wrote his supplement prescriptions with the exact dosages and times and I think he threw it some meds too. When the doctor was finished I proceeded with the script to the front desk. The staff member went into a storage room and gathered the magic pills. Approximately $500 worth of the magic pills were presented and I paid out pocket for them. Also, the office visit was not covered by my insurance. I left with my instructions and more supplements than I ever bought in one shot in my life. I faithfully took the supplements for the prescribed 30 days and returned for a follow-up. There was one catch, I did not change my diet or lifestyle at all. See, at the time opinions about nutrition varied. There was the heavy supplement approach, the food based approach and the combination approach. Luckily my teachers were great and they covered nutrition, lifestyle and supplements in good balance. So you can see when I was given a massive supplement program with the nutritional and lifestyle recommendation under-emphasized, it felt unbalanced to me. However, I was given my orders to supplement, which I did and returned for follow-up. At the follow up, I was generally the same.

During my follow-up consultation, I described having no improvement in energy, vitality, stress, etc. I was prescribed the same supplement regimen. As the doctor was again writing the script for another $500 worth of the magic pills, which by themselves provided limited, if any, benefit, I asked a most important question. "Doc, if I do not change my diet and lifestyle will these help?" His answer was funny because he say basically no, not if you don't change your lifestyle.

Then he appeared to get annoyed and said to me "What, do you want to see my nutritionist?"

I did not need to see his nutritionist, as at the time I was earning my Master's degree in Nutrition. I knew exactly what to do but I was like everyone else; I was allowing everything else in my life to become more of a priority than my health. I knew the answer to my question prior to seeing this doctor. I guess I wanted to hear it for myself.

So after spending over 2,000 bucks out of pocket, I got a good learning experience. There is no magic out there. You have to do the work. Supplements help, but only when coupled with your own proper nutrition plan. We need supplements; our food supply is not as nutritional as it once was due to processing and soil contents. The stress of a poor economy, pollution, work and family can drain your body. These points alone make the case for supplements in your routine. And if you want to achieve optimal health you need nutrients at a higher level than can be provided in your diet. But remember that your nutritional intake and dietary habits are the most important and first line of defense in health. Supplements are supplemental to your diet and should not replace proper eating. That said what should you supplement with and how often. This is where it becomes real confusing. Unfortunately, it is a jungle out there.

The Flood Gates Open

In 1994, the Dietary Supplement Health and Education Act (DSHEA), was initiated. The DSHEA defines a dietary supplement as: "...a product (other than tobacco) that is intended to supplement the diet that bears or contains one or more of the following dietary ingredients: a vitamin, a mineral, an herb or other botanical, an amino acid, a dietary substance for the use by man to supplement the diet by increasing the total daily intake, or a concentrate, metabolite, constituent, extract, or combinations of these ingredients...."

You can see how this opened up the field of supplement companies to a whole new wave of products to sell. Furthermore, supplements are regulated more like food than prescription drugs. Dietary supplements can be marketed and sold without having any product research on its safety or effectiveness. For a dietary supplement to be removed from the selves it has to be deemed unsafe. This usually occurs when enough adverse reactions are reported to the Food and Drug Administration (FDA).

So basically if a product is deemed as not causing harm or at least nothing harmful that can be tied to it you can buy it. There are so many supplements for sale all around us. From the old mom and pop nutritional stores they had when I was a kid, which I think were the best, to big chain stores, supermarkets, and the internet, it's abundant. And it appears that everyone has the magic pills, formulas or potions for sale. I remember while driving to my brother's house I was listening to a health show on the radio. As I listened, the host was taking calls and given advice. His advice was basically take his product. And the funny thing was it was just one product and the callers had a variety of ailments. Headaches take my product, toe fungus, take my product, low sex drive, take my product and give it to your wife too. I am having fun with it but you get my point. Then a caller came on the line and said she was in a recent car accident and had severe neck pain and was unable to use her arm due to numbness.

As I got mad waiting for his obvious response of taking his product and all will be well, he whiffed. He waited for a while and say I think you need to see a specialist. That probably was gut wrenching for him not to push his product but I guess sometimes the right thing hurts someone like that.

So what can you do to help yourself find quality products? The best way would be to work with a qualified health professional that can review your current situation and make prudent recommendations. I am sure that the doctor I visited had quality supplements, he just charged too much and prescribed too many (shot gun approach). However, to his defense better nutrition on my part, fewer supplements would be needed.

You must do Your Homework

If going to a professional is not an option, learn how to read. Yes read, read about ingredients and read labels. A good website to help you decide if your supplement is ok is the Natural Medicines Comprehensive Database. It can give you reports on certain supplements and ingredients. If you want to take a supplement just type it in and see what they say. Not every product is in there but most ingredients are. This resource will help you get a leg up on getting the proper knowledge on the supplements you are taking. It is always a good idea to understanding what you are putting into your body. When I was studying for my nutrition degree I was often using the Natural Medicines Comprehensive Database as a valuable resource. I believe for a small monthly fee you can get more in depth reports on supplements.

After you check with your health provider and pharmacist about possible medication interactions the next step is to check ingredient and supplement safety. That can be made clearer by checking the database. I cannot stress the point of checking with your pharmacist or health provider if you have a medical condition or are taking any medications. You should not be scared to supplement but identify any harmful interactions with your condition. Get this information from the people who deal with disease, your doctor and pharmacist, this is where the shine, crisis care. I was once in a health food store and an elderly woman asked the sales person if her husband can take supplements she was purchasing. She explained to the sales person that her husband has a heart condition. The sales person said without hesitation or viewing the product, "Sure, they are herbs and are safe." Well herbs are like natural medicine and can interact with certain medications, so be sure.

Other good resources on current supplement research that I like are Consumer Labs, the Tufts newsletter and Vitasearch. These sources provide good quality information. Subscribe to one or all to better understand what you are taken. A word of caution about research. Sometimes studies have to be reviewed by a health professional or someone qualified that can read beyond the headlines. An example could be that vitamin X, which claims to improve cardiovascular health, is unproven. This is due to a study on vitamin X and cardiac benefit showed limited benefit. Upon further review, could it be that the study had limited subjects and most had advanced heart disease, which is beyond what vitamin X is supposed to help. Pretty tough to find a good result in this case. So a detailed look is important.

After you know the safety or non-safety of the supplements you are going to take what's next. How about checking the quality of the supplements you are taking. This is very hard as there is so many products on the market. And the marketing of a lot of these products is intense. Everyone knows the names of the major brands that are promoted on most of the store shelves. Most claim to give you your life back. And forget about the radio and TV shows that preach the fountains of youth. One important way to help you identify better quality products is to look for the USP verified mark on the label. I am not saying that if a product does not have the USP mark it is a bad product. However, the United States Pharmacopeia developed a highly comprehensive and rigorous dietary supplement program to address dietary supplement quality.

After rigorous review a USP verified marked product reliably contains the products that are listed on the label with the declared strengths and amounts that are also listed. The product also will break down the ingredients and release them with in a specific time for better availability into your body. And they do not contain harmful levels of contaminants which can be found in non-tested products. The USP standards also indicates that the product has been manufactured using Good Manufacturing Practices (GMP). These GMPs are defined by the USP.

You can find of list of USP verified products on the Natural Medicines Comprehensive Database. Also, if you are working with a qualified health provider they usually have access to products that the general public does not, supposedly. I say supposedly because it seems like anything can be found on the Internet, but beware. Many companies that work exclusively with health providers have high quality products and follow strict manufacturing standards. The main jury for providers are their patients. I have seen numerous companies that only deal with health professionals, change and improve product formulations based on doctor feedback. That is a good standard to go by- *RESULTS*.

The Magnificent Seven

Now it's time to add some supplements to your healthy diet. Remember what I emphasized about nutrition – FOOD FIRST. Follow the nutritional guidelines that have been presented before you take supplements. The ideal situation is to be evaluated to see what is specifically needed in your case. The more data (lab work, hormone panels, urinalysis, etc.) on how your body is functioning the better the strategy to health. Depending on dietary and health factors, a specific nutritional supplement protocol can be used. If you feel you might need more advanced nutritional work then seek a qualified professional and go for it. If you don't need any specific work and just want a healthy edge here are my general recommendations. In my experience people do not like to take supplements. If you give them too many supplements to take on a daily basis they will eventually stop taking them. And with a solid diet you will get most of the nutrients you need from food.

The seven supplements I feel we can benefit from in no particular order are:

- **Good Quality Multi-vitamin/mineral**
- **Vitamin D3**
- **Astaxanthin**
- **Omega 3Fatty Acids/Fish Oils**
- **CoQ10**
- **Greens Drink**
- **Magnesium**

Just a couple of points on my, "The Magnificent Seven". You might be saying that your favorite supplement is not on this list. That's fine because these are my recommendation based on my experience that can give most people the best bang for their buck. If you take a supplement that is not on the list and it benefits you, go for it. If you are on a specific supplement program that is individualized to your needs then stick to it. This is a powerful, general wellness recommendation.

Also of note is you will see high dose recommendation, as opposed to the RDA or daily values. This is because the RDA's (Recommended Daily Allowances) that were first introduced in 1941 were used to combat diseases of malnutrition and vitamin/mineral deficiency. Some examples would be scurvy (vitamin C deficiency), beri-beri, (vitamin B1 deficiency) and pellagra (niacin deficiency). They worked well; today you don't hear about many cases of these types of diseases.

Today the RDA is part of the Dietary Reference Intake System. This system also includes RDI (Reference or Recommended Daily Intake), Daily Values, which appear on ingredient labels and upper tolerate limits. Many nutritionists say these limits are inadequate for optimal health.

Doctors Emanuel Cheraskin and W.M. Ringsdorf, Jr from the University of Alabama School of Medicine conducted a 15-year study that looked at the health and diets of 13,500 men and woman in different areas of the United States. One of their conclusions was: The healthiest individuals also took supplements.

Using this data on what healthy individuals consume, Alex Schauss, Ph.D developed the Suggested Optimal Nutrient Allowances (SONA).

To see how these values compare to the RDA of certain vitamins, here is a good example:

In looking at Vitamin C for example, the RDA is between 75-90 mgs, and I have seen it recommended as low as 60 mgs per day. The SONA value is 800-1000 mgs. This is the difference of having one eight ounce cup of orange juice for the RDA value, as compared to 11 cups to satisfy the SONA recommendation. Still think you don't need to supplement?

Here is a little more detail on The Magnificent Seven, with my personal dose recommendations. The dosages are what I personally take for optimal wellness. Since you are a different individual with different needs always consult with a physician or a qualified health provider before you start.

- ***Good Quality Multivitamin/ Mineral.*** This should be the first line of defense. It is recommended that every adult and child take a multivitamin daily. Taking a good multi can help you get the adequate amounts of vitamins and minerals you need to reduce the risk of chronic diseases. Word of caution: not all multivitamins are the same, so do your homework. Cheaper is not always better, nor is expensive always the answer. I recommend iron-free for males, as you don't want to overload on iron if your iron level is good. Dosage depends on product, however can be based on age, activity level and needs. As with most supplement recommendations I like to see testing done to be more accurate.

- ***Vitamin D3*** – This has been highly published in recent years with good reason. Vitamin D is beneficial in helping with bone health, immune support and dealing with certain cancers. In my experience most people have low vitamin D levels. This can be determined by measuring your serum 25-hydroxy vitamin D (25(OH)D3) level. The normal range is 32-100 ng/mL with a range of 40 -70 considered optimal. We are developed to get vitamin D from the sun. Once it hits your skin it is converted to D3. However, due to our inability to get adequate amount of sun during the day due to work, school or the environment, we become deficient. I recommend that you get your vitamin D level tested and check with your doctor before you supplement.

If your level is within the optimal ranges then you are probably doing the right thing. If you supplement to get to the optimal range start at 400-1000 IU to see how you respond. Then if you are ok with that dose you can increase it.

Dosage recommended is 4000 -5000 IU (international units) daily. However, your need will depend on test levels. If you are low you need at least 4000-5000 IU daily. If you are within the optimal range of 40-70 ng/mL, then 2000 IU's daily should help keep you there. If you are taking a good amount of vitamin D and still have low levels after a few months of supplementing you might have an absorption problem and should get tested to see if you have underlying GI issues.

- *Astaxanthin* – this is a supplement that is getting a lot of high marks lately. Many nutritional experts are touting its benefits. I just heard an expert on a radio interview discussing astaxanthin and its health riches. Astaxanthin is a member of the carotenoid family. It is a powerful antioxidant and it is what gives salmon its pinkish color. It is found in salmon as well as in Krill oil. Besides its antioxidant effect it has been used to help with infertility, improved vision and cardiovascular health.

My recommended dosage is 4-16mgs. You can get approximately 1-5mgs of astaxanthin from a serving of salmon.

- *Omega 3 fatty acids/ fish oils* – great for reducing inflammation, they are also good for nervous system, heart, joint, skin and immune system. The key is to balance your Omega 3 fatty acids with your omega 6 fatty acids. A poor diet consisting of grains, Trans fats, and processed foods will increase your omega 6's. This balancing act should be a 2-1 ration of omega 6's to omega 3's and no worse than a 6-1 ratio of omega 6's to 3's. A typical poor diet like I just mentioned can increase this ratio as high as 20-30 to 1.

Dosage recommended is 1200 mgs to 2400 mgs daily with a higher ratio of EPA (eicosapentaenoic acid) to DHA (docosahexaenoic acid).

- *CoQ10 (ubiquinol)* - is a powerful antioxidant, which is found in every cell in the body, hence the word it is derived from, ubiquitous, which means everywhere. It is important for energy utilization in the mitochondria, the powerhouse of the cells. It also deals with the biosynthesis of ATP, GTP and UTP from the foods we eat for energy. It is widely used for heart health and if someone is taking a statin drug it is a smart strategy to supplement with CoQ10. This is because to lower cholesterol a statin also lowers the pathway which produces CoQ10. The body converts CoQ10 (ubiquinone) to ubiquinol to be used for health benefits. However, as we age our ability to convert CoQ10 to ubiquinol declines. This is not a good situation for your energy level.

Dosage recommended is 100-200mg daily.

- ***Greens or Reds Drink*** – I see a lot of greens or vegetable drinks out there. There are also a good amount of reds or fruit drinks available. I presently jump start every day with my Greens drink mixed with whey or rice protein and 8 ounces of coco-nut milk. Sometimes I will use the red drink, but I usually eat a fair amount of fruits. And depending on your dietary makeup it would be wise to supplement with what you might be lacking. Now these are not fruit juices or ready- made drinks but rather are concentrated powder mixes that you combine with water, juice or in my case coconut milk. They provide high level anti-oxidant protection which can be measured by its ORAC value which stands for Oxygen Radical Absorbance Capacity. ORAC is a measurement which determines the biological antioxidant capacity in a foodstuff. These drinks can also contain proprietary blends of fiber, enzymes and probiotics.

Dosage recommended is usually one scoop depending on the product.

- ***Magnesium*** – this is an under looked at gem. Magnesium is involved in around 300 enzymatic reactions in the body. It is used for nerve and muscle health, cramping of muscles and bone health. Enough said, it is a powerful supplement.

Dosage Recommended is 400 mg per day.

These are *"The Magnificent Seven"* that I feel are a good base to get on the road to wellness. They should be used in supplement with good nutrition from your food. If you eat poorly and just try to supplement it is like putting premium gasoline in a jalopy.

It you are gung ho and want a little extra boost here are three that make it a perfect ten.

Vitamin C (Ascorbic acid) – has been known for years to help boost your immune system and provide antioxidant protection. It can help reduce the duration of cold symptoms and infections. It is needed for the biosynthesis of connective proteins, like collagen. It can also help with inflammation.

Dosage recommended is 1000-2000 mg per day. I prefer to take Vitamin C powder and if you are not use to taking large amounts of vitamin C then you can gradually titrate up from about 250-500mgs per day till you can reach optimal levels. If you get loose stools then back off a little till you normalize.

Probiotics – to help restore and repair your intestinal flora which is essential for overall health, probiotics should be taken. Probiotics are microbial components of microbial cells that improve health and well-being. They help with promoting healthy flora, preventing pathogenic bacteria to fester, reduce inflammation and help with overall gut health. The two common and powerful probiotics that are in many top products are Lactobacillus acidophilus and bifid bacterium.

Dosage is usually in the millions of cells of the probiotics that the supplement contains. This sounds like a lot but it is usually in one or two capsules. This of course can vary according to the supplement you use.

B-Complex – you should get some of you B-vitamins from your multi-vitamin and food. However, since the B's are so important for energy and overall health an extra dose can be healthful.

Dosage varies with different supplement.

One another important item I need to mention is dietary fiber, which is also called roughage or bulk. Dietary fiber contains parts of plant foods that your body can't digest or absorb. Because it is hard to break down it passes through your stomach, small intestine, and colon, then exits your body.

Benefits of a high-fiber diet can include: normalizing bowel movements, helps maintain a healthy bowel, lowers cholesterol levels, helps control blood sugar and can aid in achieving a healthy body weight.

According to the Institute of Medicine, the average daily recommendations for adults are: if you are a man age 50 or younger you need 38 grams per day. If you are over 50 you need 30 grams. Females need 25 grams if under 50 and 21 grams once they pass the big 50.

A product I like is **Barndad's Fiber DX**. I came across Fiber Dx in talking to Kurt Angle, 1996 Olympic Gold Medalist in freestyle wrestling. Kurt is also a pro wrestling superstar for TNA Impact wrestling and previously in the WWE. I heard Kurt speak at the 2011 NCAA wrestling Championships in Philadelphia on obesity and physical fitness and his message resonated. One of his recommended products is Fiber DX which can help curb your appetite and help you lose weight. More information can be found at www.barndadnutrition.com.

Also I recommend that you do a medically supervised detox program twice or three times per year. This can help you give your liver and body a break from the toxins that we have to deal with. I said it should be supervised by a qualified health provider because of the complications that can occur with detoxification. I have had patients get ill, experience severe headaches and other problems which can occur when your body is dealing with toxin elimination. Being able to monitor each patient helps increase the success rate and minimize problems.

These are my recommendations and I am sticking to it so let's roll on.

Chapter 14

GET OFF THAT COUCH AND MOVE IT

You have been consuming many statistics on health through-out this book. You should understand the difference between health and fitness. You can be a highly fit individual and have health issues. The prior few sections deal with nutritional components of wellness. If I had to pick either proper nutrition or exercise to be healthy my pick would be nutrition. That is if you only can pick one. The good news is that you don't have to pick just one. In fact, to truly be well you need proper nutrition and proper exercise. If you are going to achieve your goal of ultimate wellness or at less the best you can be, you need both. This is especially true if you are in need of some moderate body fat reduction. I see many people try to just change their nutrition, mostly drastically reduce calories, to lose weight. They often fail because without exercise to help burn calories you have to eat much less.

The hard part is that exercise is work and many of us hate to work. Complicating this fact is we are often very busy to find the time to exercise. Now that is of course a problem if you want to train like an Olympian but that is not necessary to get healthier. As you will see you can improve with exercise using very little time. Now I personally need a gym to workout. I like to do resistance training or weight lifting as my favorite form of exercise. I also use medicine balls, kettle-bells and resistance bands as supplements to my weight lifting. For me this requires a gym to accomplish and I usually workout 45 minutes to an hour. That is the way I like to go about it but you must find your way.

The key is to find your groove. Do an exercise routine you enjoy and can be consistent with. You need to change your routine every few weeks so your body can adapt. And this can be applied to any type of exercise. You can add time, resistance, change the exercise type or exercise order to adapt changes in the body. Remember to check with your physician or health provider before starting any fitness routine. Once cleared and you get over the initial soreness you will feel the blood flowing and the life returning to your limbs.

In designing your routine you have to understand and incorporate the components of fitness to be fit. You need to develop your cardio vascular system, strength, endurance, flexibility and improve your body composition (less body fat more lean muscle tissue). This is important because many people that exercise may concentrate on one or two of these areas and neglect the others.

A prime example is individuals that use walking as their only mode of fitness. Walking is probably the easiest and less expensive exercise you can do. Just go out the front door and go. However, I have seen many walkers that neglect their strength and flexibility. This can cause major problems. You can solve this by adding some flexibility and strength training to get a more complete fitness program. Another component to practice is stability. If your body is not stable during important positions and movements you will get hurt. This can be accomplished by using more functional movements in you exercises. With proper instruction, stability balls and balance boards are great to improve stability.

Time is a major problem with people today as everyone seems to be too busy or in a hurry. One day as I finished working on a patient I went into the waiting area to go get some water from the water cooler. As my head was turned toward the cooler I heard the front door behind me open and close. As I looked I realized that my patient basically followed right behind me, passing the front desk and verbally scheduled her next appointment with my staff on the fly. She could not even stop for a second to make the appointment she just did it on her way out never missing a step. That made me realize it is a go- go world. If this sounds like you, let me introduce you to high intensity interval training or HIIT.

High intensity interval training is what it sounds like. It is a specific training program which uses very high intensity exercise in a series of intervals. It is designed to alternate between bouts of exercise and rest intervals. The mode of exercises that can be used is variable. These can be sprints, cycling, weights, bands, kettle-bells, or body weight exercises. Whatever you enjoy and will be consistent with. This is a very demanding workout designed to push your anaerobic capacity (without oxygen) and you will be exhausted after it. With that being say you need to check with your medical provider to make should you are fit enough to try this. Couch potatoes relax for a moment I will get to you later, but keep this type of training in the back of your mind for future use. Once you decide on what exercise or exercises you are going to do you can begin. I personally like a program that uses some resistance training.

Resistance training can help increase your bone mineral density which is important for battling osteoporosis. It also strengthens muscles and joints and improves posture. Using light dumbbells, kettle bells and resistance bands are great for HIIT.

When I was in a fitness class in school the instructor put us through a great workout using intervals. We used 3 pound dumbbells for woman and 10 pounds for men. Your weight selection is all individualized. We would exercise all out for around 20-30 seconds and rest or stretch for about 10-15 seconds. These cycles were repeated for a 15-20 minute workout. The exercises were varied and used most of your body. Examples were squats with presses, lunges and presses, variations of rowing movements, push-ups, etc. You can use many different exercises.

You can be very simple if you like — a basic treadmill or stationary bike is just fine. The main key is, you want to exercise all-out for a predetermined time and rest after the exercise for a predetermined time— This is one cycle. Repeat your cycles till you reached the total time for your workout.

In my example, we performed a dumbbell exercise like a squat and press for about 30 seconds and rested for about 15 seconds—that is a 45 second cycle. That is tough and I had to pace myself for a few workouts till I was able to go hard. We continued these 45 second cycles using different exercises till we reached a 15-20 minute session. Your sessions should last around 20 minutes or less and should not be performed on consecutive days. Your body needs to recover and if you overdue it you can get hurt. Start very slow with shorter exercise intervals, longer rest and shorter session duration. Built yourself up and monitor your improvement.

If you really want more bang for your buck in the shortest possible time, how does four minutes sound? That's right just four minutes a day, three times a week can help you can help you get fit. It can also help your burn fat. It's the Tabata training method, which was developed by Izumi Tabata, PhD at the National Institute of Fitness and Sport in Tokyo, Japan.

The guidelines for this four minutes of glory or torture are:
- Decide you mode of exercise, cardio, weights, etc.
- Warm up for 5-10 minutes to increase blood flow
- Exercise all out for 20 seconds, then rest for 10 seconds
- Repeat the 20 seconds of exercise-10 seconds rest cycles for four minutes.

For most of you this type of training is too intense at the moment. I say at the moment because this should be the goal of most of you. Imagine what your fitness level would be after you apply the HITT or Tabata methods as your exercise. I understand this may not be it the stars for some of you. An injury or condition might make it more difficult. Or you might just be a couch potato and going from 0 to 100 miles per hour might be too much for you to handle.

Most people can incorporate a walking program into their lives. The street and parks are free. Just go out the front door and do it. You can add variety and difficulty by changing you mileage, add hills if possible or pick up the pace. It can help keep your bodyweight down and improve the ole ticker. Walking will not help too much with strength and flexibility, but as mentioned earlier they can be added.

What happens if you are one of the many people that just does not have the time. You rise early and get home late and your day is a blur. Well listen up. If you sit most of your day you are harming yourself. We mentioned this earlier how a sedentary lifestyle ruins your health. Even if you workout intensively you still have a sedentary lifestyle.

One of the things to do is try not to sit so long. If you can move more that would help. I try not to sit and do my notes. I have a computer tablet and stand while I do notes as much as possible. Another thing to do is to incorporate some exercise while on the job. Having a chair and desk with some small dumbbells is all you need for my "FITSIT" exercise program. This is to be performed twice a day, once in the morning and afternoon. You can get fit while you sit. Using the following eight exercises daily can help you improve your fitness.

- *Chair squat* – sit at the edge of your chair and place both feet on the ground. Stick your chest out to improve posture, tighten your stomach and glutes (buttocks) and stand up. Return to chair and repeat 10-20 times.
- *Chair Squat with Weights* – holding a dumbbell at your sides (5 pounds for woman and 10 pounds for men) perform the chair squat as before. Repeat 10-20 times.
- *Rotate and Reach* – Sit up straight at the edge of your chair, then slowly rotate (twist) to the right and reach both arms up and back. Repeat to the left. Repeat 5 times each side.
- *Seated Bicep Curls* – using the dumbbells you used for the *squat with weights* exercise, sit at the edge of your chair with the weights at your side. Your arms should be straight with palms facing in toward your body. Slowing bend your elbow and raise the weights up to your shoulders at the same time. Your palms should rotate toward the ceiling when rising the weight and should rotate inward toward the body when returning to the starting position. Repeat 10 times. If your chair arms are in the way you can perform the exercise standing.
- *Overhead Presses* – using the same dumbbells, bring them to your shoulders. Keep good posture with your chest out and stomach nice and tight. With your head facing straight slowly raise the weights overhead. Do not arch or round your back. Return to shoulders and repeat 10 times.
- *Lateral Shoulder Raises* – Sit at the edge of your chair in good posture with your chest out and head facing straight ahead. Take your dumbbells and lift them out to the side in an arcing

motion to your shoulder level. Do not raise above your shoulders Once again if your chair arms are in the way you can perform this exercise standing. Repeat 10 times. Start with light weight like 1-3 pounds for woman and 5 pounds for men. As you get stronger slowly lift more, but no more than 5 pounds for woman and 10 pounds for men. This will help protect your shoulder joints.

- ***Single Leg Stand and Raise***- This exercise requires that you stand at your desk. You may have to balance yourself by holding on to the edge of your desk or a door knob. Start by standing up and raising your right leg with your knee bend to 90 degrees. You will be standing on your left leg with your right knee flexed to 90 degrees and your right foot parallel to the ground. Hold this position for 15 seconds. Then while maintaining your single leg stance bring your knee and leg back so that your thigh is in line with your body and your foot is perpendicular to the floor. Hold this position for 15 seconds. Repeat with left leg. Repeat this cycle 2 more times for a total of 3 cycles.

- ***Abdominal Hold*** – Sit up straight with good posture and draw in your stomach. Try to imagine getting your belly button to your spine. This is not abdominal bracing used for core exercises. You are basically sucking in your gut and holding. Hold 15-30 and remember to breath. Repeat 3 times.

This whole routine should take you less than 10 minutes. As you become fitter you can increase the number of repetitions or time to make it more challenging. So skip the coffee and donuts and FITSIT.

Another excuse is that I can't afford a gym. I presented a few very good and convenient exercise programs. You can work out quickly so time is not an excuse. You can get fit at your desk so working all the time is not an excuse. If you prefer the gym like I do that's fine. I have been a gym rat my whole life and my fitness levels equals to my gym time. However, money and time can be an issue.

Twenty years ago I would say you would be up a creek without a paddle. Home workout equipment left much to be desired. If a piece of equipment was good enough to get a good work out it was too expensive.

Nowadays there are some very good home exercise systems that are good quality and affordable. I personally use three different systems that I can use in between patients for some exercise or when I can't get to the gym. The three I use are the Rack Workout, TRX Suspension training and the Tower 200. Why do I use three systems? Because I get bored easily and like variety. The Rack and TRX are good for body weight exercises. That is a problem for most of us, we can't lift our body. Ever see people get out of a chair or pick something up. Our movement patterns are poor and we have too many weaknesses. The Tower 200 by Body by Jake fits on your door and is an efficient pulley resistance system. It has three levels of resistance on each pulley. The tension is 25, 35, and 40 pounds respectively. This is important as even a beginner can get a workout using the light tension. The pulleys are set up in high and low position so a variety of exercises can be used. I use it mostly for rowing exercises and rotational movements. All these systems come with complete workouts at different skill levels and are priced around 200 bucks or lower. So now there are no excuses.

Chapter 15

OH MY ACHING BACK

It is fitting that the end of this book deals with the initial motivation for writing it: BACK PROBLEMS. I have spent the last 20 plus years dealing with this issue. I have dealt with patients needing a regular spinal tune up (chiropractic adjustment), as well as, ones that came into my office by ambulance. From grannies that could barely rise from a chair to world class athletes. I have read, studied and observed many aspects of this saga and read my lips, I have come up with the following conclusion. YOU MUST TAKE CARE OF YOUR SPINE FOR YOUR ENTIRE LIFE, PERIOD.

This occurs from childhood till they put you in the ground. I marvel at dentistry and the way the dental profession educated the public years ago on the importance of dental health. When I was a child you rarely visited the dentist. You hated it and after a while your parents would only take you if you had pain. Sounds like a crisis care approach to me. Remember Austin Powers' dental issues during the movie "Austin Powers, International Man of Mystery." The 1960s dental programs didn't seem up to stuff.

I used to brag about how I spent my teenage years rarely needing a dentist. This was until I saw one at age 21 and I was told that I had the beginning of gum disease. This became a problem for the next several years. I still could not get it through my thick head that I needed to take care of my teeth. The only time I really did any regular dental visits in my twenties was for cosmetic reasons and some cleanings, but regular home care, besides a once daily brushing, was limited. I did not even know how to floss. It did not happen for me till my gum disease got so bad that I was looking at some pretty hefty dental bills if I did not change my ways. Like magic, I have seen the light and have since brushed, flossed, gargled and attended to regular cleanings, which to date have given me a rather benign set of choppers and gums.

What does this have to do about your back? Remember the premise of this book is to change your attitude. The dental profession has done a marvelous job over the years since I was a kid educating the public on the importance of dental care. I have difficulty in referring patients to my dentist because everyone seems to have one. The funny thing is that after all the cleanings, brushing and flossing if you live long enough your teeth decay and you get false ones. Answer yourself this. You can live pretty good with false teeth, correct? Talk to someone who has a chronic debilitating back problem and see how they are living. My guess is they would rather have the dentures. Isn't it time that we start to take proactive care of our spine just like we do our teeth, hair, nails and even our cars.

Back pain is an epidemic in my view. Approximately 80% of the population will report some type of back pain in their lifetime. I have. Did you experience back pain in your lifetime yet? There are many causes of back pain from injuries that can damage spinal structure like sports injuries, auto accidents and falls. Also certain conditions like scoliosis, osteoarthritis, rheumatoid arthritis, infections, tumors to name a few can debilitate a back. However, I want to concentrate on prevention of back problems by helping you built a healthy back. Most of the back problems that I see are mechanical in nature. This means in my terms, that your spinal alignment and movement is not optimal and slowly but surely you are placing undo and uneven stresses to your spinal structures. This can be caused by poor posture, reduced joint and muscle flexibility, altered spinal alignment and deconditioned muscles. We place our bodies in unhealthy positions through- out the day which create havoc on the spine. We sit too long, stand too much and bend and twist incorrectly. I call this dilemma ***"Ergonomic Spinal Syndrome"*** or E.S.S. The way we work and live negatively affects our spinal health.

To understand "E.S.S" we first have to take a basic spinal anatomy lesson. First, your spine has three basic regions. The cervical or neck region, you're thoracic, which runs from the base of the neck to the top of your lumbar or low back region. Think of your thoracic spine as the part that contains your ribs. As mentioned your lumbar or low back region is at the bottom. You also have a large bone beneath the lumbar region called the "sacrum." The sacrum is the result of the fusion of several vertebra. At the end or just below the sacrum is the coccyx. This is what is called your tailbone. Also of note is that above the cervical spine we have your skull. This is important as we will see because head position is so crucial.

As we look into each specific region of the spine you see they have some differences. The cervical or neck region consists of seven individual vertebrae. The curve in the cervical region is lordotic, which means that there is an anterior (front) convexity in the curvature. This lordosis is also present in the lumbar spine.

The thoracic spine is the spinal region that has rib attachments. In this region there are twelve individual vertebrae. The curvature in the thoracic spine is the opposite of the cervical and lumbar spines. Thoracic curvature is called a "kyphotic" which bows the spine outward. This type of curvature can become pronounced and appears as a hump back. Remember the hunchback of Notre Dame?

The low back region is called the "lumbar spine". In this area there are five individual vertebrae. In combining these three regions there are 24 vertebrae, barring any fusion of vertebra or congenital factors. The important factors to understand in the spine are these 24 vertebrae have to have proper movement and alignment.

Let's talk about alignment for a moment. Your spine should have nicely lined up curves looking from the side and should be straight from the front and back.

Very simply, if I am looking at someone's standing posture I like to evaluate them from the side, front and back. Some practitioners will measure spinal alignment with computerized programs or with x-rays. I will do this too on certain cases but basically I do a visual evaluation. From the front or anterior view, I imagine a plumb line from the top of the person's head and run it through their nose to the middle of the sternum or mid thorax. From there, I look at it through the umbilicus and middle of the pubic bone to the floor. Basically it is right through the center of the body. From this view I can compare the right and left sides. I look to see if the head is centered properly and the shoulders are even. I check their pelvic alignment and evaluate their knees and feet.

From the back or posterior view, I still look at the right and left side for comparison but I also look at the shoulder blades to make sure they are not winging or protruding away from the body (sticking out). I will also look at the back of the ankle, basically the Achilles tendon to see if it bows inward which could indicate a foot pronation problem. In the side or lateral view, I run the imaginary plumb line from the center of the head through the ear and middle of the shoulder. From there I run it through the center of the hip and knee joint and just in front of the lateral malleolus (the big bump on the outside of your ankles). From the side, I look to see if the head is centered over the shoulders properly.

Forward head translation is a common postural problem and with many of us constantly working on computers and text messaging it appears to be getting worse. I also look to see if the lordotic curves in the neck and low back are aligned properly and if the body is not shifting forward or backward. In addition to looking at postural alignment, while doing the evaluation I also look at muscle tone. It is very common to see muscle imbalances that can be created by faulty posture, or overworking a muscle. Ever see someone that is in a slumped posture possibly from years of computer work.

The muscles in the front of their body might be shortened or tight and the back muscles could be overstretched. As the years go by this posture can become permanent.

If you have ideal posture it will help minimize stress and strain on your structural tissues, like muscles, joints, ligament and discs. The problem I forgot to mention is posture is not just how you stand but how you move, sit, bend, reach, etc.

I routinely ask patients to walk down my office hallway to watch the way they walk. There is a lot of biomechanical information a practitioner can get from watching someone walk. A common flaw I see is that most people walk with a short stride. This means that they do not extend their legs backward or bring them forward enough as they walk. It almost appears that they have a belt around their thighs as they take short steps. This can mean possibly some joint restrictions or muscle dysfunction.

To check to see if someone has problems with their joints and muscle I look at ROM (range of motion) to the spinal regions, as well as the upper and lower extremities. The body works together and should be evaluated as such. It is amazing how much information is missed if you just concentrate on the area of complaint. It is not uncommon to injury your ankle or leg and if not corrected you can develop problems elsewhere. I have seen patients develop problems on the other side of the body from the site of original complaint.

This is common in athletes and active people. I have seen this numerous times considering by heavy involvement with athletic injuries. A couple of examples which come to mind are a marathon runner came to see me about right hip pain while running. During evaluation I had him run for a couple of minutes on a treadmill which caused hip pain. As he ran, I noticed that his left arm was not swinging properly as compared to his right arm. He had no known injury to the arm and only complained of hip pain. I worked mostly on his left shoulder to reduce the restrictions and muscle imbalances. Once he got back on the treadmill his arms moved more evenly and his hip pain was gone.

The second example was a high level tri-athlete I evaluated for shoulder pain. In his case I did not have the luxury of watching him run on a treadmill so I had to rely on posture, ROM and functional testing. Functional testing is similar postural assessment only during movement. I have the patient perform movements to see if they can do them properly or have imbalances side to side. I typically look at squatting movement, one leg squats, how they balance, lunge forward, backward and to the side and other various shoulder and upper extremity movements.

While evaluating this athlete his ROM and movements were good. He did have some pain and mild weakness on manual muscle testing in the shoulder. Manual muscle testing is another analysis tool used to evaluate muscle function which is a little too complex to explain for this book. However, on a more simple note, when I looked at his posture he had an elevated shoulder. In other words one of his shoulders from the front view was sticking up higher than the other. This was in the front standing position. Remember I said that posture is not just standing. Knowing that in a triathlon there is a lot of running in races and in training, I asked him to sit down while I re-checked his posture. As he sat down his shoulders leveled indicating to me that his problem could possibly be lower extremity related (feet, ankle, knees, etc,). In evaluating his feet one of his arches was dropped. This is not uncommon and he then said to me that he was also having mild foot pain. I suggested an arch support might help. He said he was already getting one from another sports doctor who also picked this flaw up. This is great doctors working together on the same page. I then put a sample arch support under his foot and re-tested his muscle strength in the shoulder. The pain was gone and strength returned.

It at times seems to the layperson and even some doctors that problems have to be linear. Especially in dealing with spinal and extremity problems. They think where it hurts is the only issue. That might be the case with some recent or acute problems. You twist an ankle or hurt your back lifting something it has to be originated where it hurts right? Suppose you twisted your ankle because your ankle joint was too tight due to an old hip injury that was not properly fixed. Or you hurt your back because your core muscles are weak and your poor back has to do all the work. Proper alignment, muscle balance, stability and flexibility are all important if you want to avoid back and joint problems. Basically more balance is needed if you want fewer problems. Speaking of back problems, I hope you did notice I did not mention any specific back problems. By now after reading this book you should know that this is about health and prevention not crisis. You all know their names. I hear them every day from patients that are in crisis. My goal is spinal wellness so we as a nation can reduce these back problems with proper education.

In my opinion in dealing with spinal and joint problems many can be avoided. I understand that trauma injuries are a different breed. Whether it is from an auto, work or sports injury they are managed differently. However, the blueprint still has to be followed if you are able. So how do you develop a healthy back in the first place? Well you have to know your enemy, E.S.S. That's right *"**Ergonomic Spinal Syndrome**,"* like I mentioned earlier. Remember we went over how important good posture and alignment is? Remember how poor posture can affect your muscles, joints, discs, ligaments, etc? It can cause excessive stress and strain on your spine and joints.

Everyday your body has to deal with ergonomic stress factors assaulting your spine and joints. Positions that we assume on a daily basis cause increased pressure to our intervertebral disc. Research has shown that simple activities like sitting and standing while bending forward can increase your intradiscal pressure. Basically the load on the intervertebral disc increases.

Also when you stand up from a chair there is an increase in disc pressure. When we lift a 20 kilogram object disc pressure is high. If you take that same 20 kilogram object and lift it bent over with rounded shoulders or away from your body your disc pressure will increase further.

These are just a few of the positions that can stress you back. What about all the positions we are in all day? Many will mess up your alignment and stress your spine. We bend, twist, stand, drive, sit all the time. What can be done to help you get a healthy back and defeat E.S.S. I like to handle E.S.S with a three prong approach. First correct the ergonomic part. This is easy once you correct your postural stress positions. Then you have to work on lifestyle changes like we have been talking about all throughout this book. Next you have to do some exercises to help stabilize your spine and support your body.

ERGONOMIC CORRECTION TIPS:

- When using a computer your monitor should be slightly below eye level and straight ahead. Your screen should be about an arm's length away and your forearms should be resting on the desk at about a 90 degree angle of the elbow with wrist relaxed and neutral.
- While sitting you should have a good chair where your feet should reach the ground and your thighs positioned at about 90 degrees or parallel to the floor. You should be able to maintain good postural alignment as we mentioned before. Use a rolled up towel

or lumbar support to maintain your lumbar curve. Avoid slouching or bending forward too much and sit at between 90 to 135 degrees. Research has shown that leaning back into about 135 degrees reduces back strain. However, I recommend you vary your position from time to time. Lean back too much can bring your chin to your chest and stress the cervical spine.

- Limit or avoid wearing high heels or any kind of platform shoes for long periods of time. This puts pressure on your back. I used to wear cowboy boots a lot when I was younger, like an urban cowboy thing, and felt how it strains the back.

- Don't sit on a wallet. It throws your pelvis out of alignment. If also gives the pick pockets a nice target.

- Get good quality sleep. Make sure your pillow is proper size. It should maintain your neck posture and curves. There are many cervical pillows out there as well as mattresses to help with sleep. I do not recommend any specific brands because these items can be pricey. Obviously a mattress cost more than a pillow but I hate to see you waste money. I used to recommend certain mattresses, but when people did not like what they bought they would get angry with me. Same with pillows to a lesser extent. Unfortunately this is trial and error as no two spines are alike and I have to be honest with you.

LIFESTYLE TIPS:
- Maintain an ideal body weight- you can't imagine how many times I have a patient come in and tell me they gained weight and hurt their back. I went over an anti-inflammation nutritional program to help with this. Re-read it if you have to.

- Work on your posture- To help with posture I teach patients proper ergonomics as I mentioned before. Also, I use specific chiropractic adjustments to free up joint restrictions and improve alignment. Specific exercises are then prescribed to strengthen muscles and increase ROM.

- Exercise, Exercise, Exercise – I have given you some easy and convenient exercises previously in this book. I will give you my favorite back ones soon but be more active. Whether you join a gym or start to walk outside, be active.

- Get a good chiropractor or therapist – one who deals with postural stresses. Most practitioners realize the importance of posture and how it stresses your body, so there are no shortages of good people out there. It's funny, my profession has been talking about spinal alignment and how it affects your health for years. Now it appears everyone is talking about. At least that is what I see when I go to seminars conducted by different disciplines. Welcome to the club.

DOC H's BACK BUILDER'S:

First I want to mention that before you start with any exercise routine or activity you need to be cleared by your medical doctor or orthopedist if that are any joint problems. Also, once cleared you need to warm up for a few minutes to get the blood flowing. Walking or a stationary bike would be fine. Just break a light sweat. Next you need to stretch the whole body. There is plenty of resources on stretching. If you are gung ho I recommend yoga or Pilates. However, gentle stretching is all that is required for these exercises because you will start out very easy. For those of you that have persistent trigger points or muscle knots you can use a tennis ball or form roller to work the kinks out prior to exercise.

WARNING, like trying to learn more on stretching use other resources to perform these properly. I recommend a Google search on gentle stretching routines, myofascial release with tennis balls, form rollers, etc. You can find plenty of information on the internet and YouTube to demonstrate the proper performance of these techniques. Just make sure they are being taught by a qualified professional. If flexibility or muscle problems become persistent see if your chiropractor or therapist is trained in soft tissue therapy and can help. Once ready the Back Builders are as follows:

<u>THE PLANK</u> – this is a basic exercise to help improve your core strength and stability.

- Begin belly down with your forearms and toes on the floor.

- Rise up keeping your torso straight and rigid and your body in a straight line from head to your feet. Do not sag down or bend upward.
- Look at the floor and hold this position for 10-15 seconds to start.
- Comfortably work up to 2- 3 sets of 45 or 60 seconds without deviating from the proper position.

To make the Plank more challenging try the following:

- Start in the same position as above belly down with your fore-arms and toes on the floor.
- Slowly raise one leg 5-8 inches off the floor while maintaining a rigid core position.
- Hold for a two count and lower your leg slowly to the floor.
- Repeat this step with the other leg for one rep.
- • Perform about 2-3 sets of 10-15 reps.

Another variation would be to lift your arm as described below:

- Start in the same position as above.
- Shift your weight to your right forearm.
- Extend your left arm straight out in front of you lined up with your body.
- Hold this position for 3 seconds while keeping a tight core.
- Bring your arm back to starting position. Switch to the right arm and repeat for one rep.
- Do 2-3 sets of 10-15 reps.

If you have difficulty with this exercise you can make it easier by performing the movement on your hands, rather than on your elbows. If you still cannot achieve this position don't worry you can do a straight arm plank against the wall. Just keep the spine and head straight and tighten your muscles.

QUADRUPED- this exercise is also a basic core stability move. It also evaluates any side deviations of the shoulders and hips. If one arm or leg raises up higher or lower than the other and imbalance is noted and needs to be corrected.

- Begin on your hands and knees. Place your hands directly in line below your shoulders. Align your head and neck with your back. Do not raise your head or lower it below your straight back position.

- Tighten your abdominal muscles as to brace them.
- Raise your right arm up off the floor and reach straight ahead. Hold this position for a count of three. Lower your right arm and repeat the same movement with your left arm. Perform 3-5 reps.
- Next from the starting position raise your right leg off the floor. Tighten your trunk muscles for stability and balance. Hold this position for a count of three. Lower your right leg and repeat the same movement with your left leg. Perform 3-5 reps.
- Next from the starting position you will lift one arm and the opposite leg at the same time. Then repeat with the other extremities. Example of this would be to raise your left arm and your right leg at the same time. Return to starting position then repeat with your right arm and left leg. Hold these positions for a count of three and perform 3-5 reps.

STABILITY BALL WALL SQUATS - I love this exercise. It is a great way to work your legs and posture if you do it correctly. It also helps with hip joint mobility. Having strong and enduring legs and good hip function will help take the stress off the lower back so this is a biggie.

- First you need a stability ball. They are those big exercise balls you see at gyms or sports medicine clinics. You can purchase one fairly inexpensive at your local sporting goods store. They also can be used for a variety of different exercises and usually come with a exercise manual.
- General size guidelines are as follows: if your height is less than 4 feet, 6 inches you would use a 30cm. ball. If you are between 4 feet six inches and five feet you can use a 45 cm. ball. From 5 feet to 5 feet and 5 inches a 55 cm. ball can be used. If you are 5 feet 6 inches tall to 6 feet 2 inches tall you can use a 65cm. This seems to be the most common ball I see being used. A 75 cm. ball is used for anyone over 6 feet 2 inches tall.
- If you are not experienced in using a stability ball get some help and always use it by a safe area in case you lose your balance. Proper footwear like sneakers or gym shoes is required.

- To begin the exercise here is the starting position.
- Place the stability ball against a wall and gently lean your back against it. The position of the ball should be into the small of your back, making contact with your tailbone, lower and middle back. Your feet should be positioned approximately 6 - 12" out in front of your body with your feet hip-width apart with toes facing forward or with a slight turned out position.
- Next pull your shoulders blades down and backward. Don't allow your lower back to pull away from the ball. Gently lean back into the ball while shifting your weight into your heels. Position your hands on the front of your thighs or across your chest.
- As you begin to downward squat inhale and keep your tailbone, low and mid-back against the ball as you begin to bend your knees. Lower your body and push back with your hips. This allows them to drop under the ball. The ball will slide down the wall with you as you lower your body. Do not move the feet. Keep your knees in line with your 2nd toe. Continue to lower yourself until your thighs align parallel to the floor or above if you feel challenged. Hold this position for a second or two.
- As you start to come up, exhale and slowly push your body up away from the floor. Extend your hips to allow them to get underneath your body. Continue to push upward, returning to your starting position. Repeat for 1-3 sets of 10-15 reps.
- Some good pointers to help you develop good squatting form. Try to emphasize dropping your hips down and slightly under the ball. Avoid driving your knees down and forward as this will place excess stress on the knees.

The last exercise requires the use of kettlebells to be performed properly. Kettlebells have their origin in Russia and look like a cannonball with a handle. They come in different weight ranges just like traditional weights. They are usually measured in kilograms, but there are some variations that come in pounds. The "King of Russian Kettlebells" is Pavel Tsatsouline. His is a complete master and has trained many in this art worldwide. He has a website, www.dragondoor.com where you can find out more information. Kettlebells can be pricey but are worth the investment. If money is an issue and for many it is you can shop around the internet or sporting goods stores for cheaper versions. Start with very light ones and work up. In my office I have patients use very light 5 to 10 pounds kettlebells to start. I recommend you find a good certified kettlebell instruct to check your form and help avoid injury. I attended a workshop taught by a friend of mine, Phil Ross of HoHoKus, NJ and could not believe how aligned and strong my body felt.

SUMO SQUAT WITH KETTLEBELL – this exercise is great for developing strength and mobility in the legs, hips and lower back muscles. For these kettlebell exercises first get the movements down with no weight. Once you are comfortable with the movements, start out very light, 5-10 pounds for woman and 10-15 pounds for men. As mentioned earlier, also check with your medical physician before beginning this or any exercise program.

- To start position yourself in a straddle stance with the feet slightly wider than the shoulders. Your toes should be pointing outward slighty. Hold a single kettlebell with both hands placed in front of your body. Use a pronated grip (palms facing the body).
- Slowly squat down while leaning slightly forward from the waist with your head up. Move downward until the upper legs are parallel the ground.
- Return to the starting position and repeat. Start at one set of 5-10 reps and work up to 2-3 sets of 10-15 reps.
- Some safety points: Remember to try to maintain good posture and not to hunch forward.
- Make sure at the end of each repetition your shoulders, knees, and balls of the feet should be aligned.
- Always keep your heels on the ground and back straight throughout the exercise.
- Always perform this exercise at a slow tempo. Do not allow the legs to lower beyond parallel to the ground. Doing this would increase the stress on the knees.

TEASER EXERCISE:

KETTLEBELLS SWINGS – another great kettlebell exercise but be careful. I recommend some coaching on this one with a certified instructor. This requires some coordination and timing so easy does it. This is such a great overall exercise that I recommend everyone starts to do it. However, if you have bad technique you can get hurt and that would defeat the purpose of this book. So your homework is to learn this exercise and do it correctly. HINT: GOOGLE IT

Well there are some of my favorites. I could have listed many more but that would complicate things. This is just the start of your journey. ASSESS, ORGANIZE, BE PATIENT, AND GO HARD FOR IT.

Yours in Strength and Health
DOC HALEY

BLUEPRINT FOR HEALTH : DOC HALEY'S

PYRAMID OF POWER GUIDELINES

The pyramid of power utilizes the main parts of the "Impatient Nation" to help give you a blueprint for success. Remember everyone is an individual and our goals might be different. The ultimate goal should be to radically improve your overall health. Before you begin the pyramid you should have a good grasp of what was presented in this book. I have covered a lot of specific information on many different aspects of being well. You should have been following the HALEYHEALTH action steps at the end of each chapter in Parts one, two and three. You should now be able to understand the recommendations and routines in Part four. To begin the pyramid let's look at each step from the bottom up.

YOU
NOW
HAVE THE
THE POWER
TO SUCCEED
CONGRATS!

Continue an anti-inflammatory diet

Participate in an activity or exercise program that
includes all or most of the fitness components
covered in the *The Impatient Nation*

Add the *"Magnificent Seven"* to your nutrition
while slowly reducing calories per day by 500

Perform the *"FITSIT"* program while at work & incorporate the *"Back Builders"* at home

Work on improving posture with the *"Ergonomic Tips"*

Improve your sleep & work on reducing stress

Start with one anti-inflammatory meal per day & work up to all daily meals. Drink MORE water

Get a check up with your physician before starting any new exercise & nutrition regimen

PYRAMID BASE:

- At the bottom of the pyramid you are first asked to get a physical exam for your physician. This has been stressed throughout the "Impatient Nation" and is strongly recommended before you start.
- Next start with exchanging one regular meal that you eat per day with a total anti-inflammatory one. If you change your eating habits too quickly you might quit. Over the next week try to eat two anti-inflammatory meals per day. Continue this till you are eating an anti-inflammatory diet.
- Increase your pure water intake. Substitute water with the drinks that you were drinking prior to changing to an anti-inflammatory diet like soda, dairy and sugary drinks.
- Review the tips on getting proper sleep and how to reduce your stress level. Also, not mentioned in the pyramid but should be a no brainer is you must work hard to eliminate any bad health habits, like smoking, excessive drinking, etc.

- Improve you posture be using the ergonomic tips presented. Gradually begin doing the BACK BUILDER exercises that were presented. These can be difficult in the beginning and you should have an exercise specialist or health professional instruct you on the proper technique. Perform 3-4 times per week.
- Finish off the bottom of the pyramid with performing the FITSIT program at work. This program can be performed twice daily, once in the morning and once in the afternoon. Perform 3-5 days per week. However, start out at once daily for 3 alternating days per week and see how your body responses.
- This part of the pyramid should take 2-4 weeks to adapt to. After that time advance to the Pyramid Center.

PYRAMID CENTER:

- Now that you are eating better you can start to add basic supplementation with the "Magnificent Seven".
- If you are trying to lose body fat gradually start to reduce your calorie intake per day. I like to see a reduction of at least 500 calories per day. Remember you will be eating more food once you stick to the anti-inflammatory guideline. However, your food choices will be naturally lower in calories.
- I also like you to start to practice food combining that was mentioned in Part four and try to spread you meals out to 3.5 to 4.5 hours between feeding. If you have to have something to eat between feedings have an anti-inflammatory snack like fruit or nuts. Also you should drink water or organic teas.
- Now you can begin to exercise with a structured program. Chose an activity that you enjoy. The components of fitness are detailed in this book but the big three for me are: Strength, Endurance and Flexibility. So if you like to walk or play tennis it might improve your endurance and flexibility somewhat. However, you would need to work on your strength. If you like to lift weights you still need to work on endurance and flexibility if not addressed.

- Once you are eating an anti-inflammatory diet and your health has improved you want to continue with a well-balanced nutritional program.

TOP OF THE PYRAMID

- Congratulations you have climbed the pyramid. You have proven to yourself and others that you have to power to succeed. Go enjoy your life.

CONCLUSION

One afternoon a very nice gentleman entered my office for treatment. This individual was in his mid-sixties and brought with him a laundry list of ailments. His list consisted of back pain, sciatica, knee pain, arthritis, diabetes, high cholesterol and blood pressure to name on few. He was also morbidly obese and could hardly walk without his knees buckling in. As I did my history he went through a long list of doctors that he seen throughout his life. What was interesting is that each and every doctor he claimed was no good. They were considered no good in his eyes because he always had problems they could not resolve. From back and knee problems to Type 2 diabetes no one could help. I recognized some of the doctors he went to and they were tops in their field. As he continued to complain I realized I would probably be added to his list of failed doctors.

I saw that he was starting to heavily see doctors well over thirty years ago in his thirties. I began to ask him about his lifestyle. I wanted to know if he ever exercised or ate right in the past or just started to fall apart in recent years. He told me he never exercised or cared about his weight. As I asked why, he told me he did not believe in that stuff. I then asked why, and he said "no doctor ever told me about that stuff." There was my answer. Not that any doctor's advice would have changed this person because he was all too typical. The blame game is rampart and it can only be stopped by personal responsibility. It begins with you the person in the mirror.

Yours in Strength and Health
Doc Haley

RESOURCES

Dr. Haley's Information: I can be reached at:
Dr. Robert J. Haley
Haley Chiropractic
528 Valley Brook Avenue
Lyndhurst, NJ 07071
201-531-9400
Website: www.haleyhealth.com

Chiropractic Organizations:
American Chiropractic Association
1701 Clarendon Boulevard
Arlington, VA 22209
Phone: 703-276-8800
Fax: 703-243-2593
http://www.acatoday.org

International Chiropractic Association
6400 ARLINGTON BLVD., STE. 800
FALLS CHURCH, VA 22042
800-423-4690
703-528-5000
Fax 703-528-5023
http://www.chiropractic.org

American Chiropractic Board of Sports Physicians (ACBSP)
103 S 6th Street, Estherville, IA 51334
+1 712 362 8860Telephone:
+1 712 362 8609FAX:
http://www.acbsp.com

Association of New Jersey Chiropractors
3121 Route 22 East, Suite 302
Branchburg, NJ 08876
Phone 908-722-5678
Fax 908-722-5677
http://anjc.info

Nutritional Organizations:
AMERICAN COLLEGE OF NUTRITION
300 S. Duncan Ave. Ste. 225
Clearwater, FL 33755
Telephone: (727) 446-6086
Fax: (727) 446-6202
http://www.americancollegeofnutrition.org

CBCN
Chiropractic Board of Clinical Nutrition
1170 Emerald Sound Blvd
Oak Point, TX 75068
(561) 402-1596
(866) 929-0361 Fax
http://www.cbcn.us

Certification Board for Nutrition Specialists
4707 Willow Springs Rd, Suite 203
La Grange, IL 60525
Phone: (202) 903-0267
Fax: (888) 712-1450
http://cbns.org

ISSN - International Society of Sports Nutrition
4511 NW 7th Street
Deerfield Beach FL 33442
http://www.sportsnutritionsociety.org

The National Weight Control Registry
Brown Medical School/The Miriam Hospital
Weight Control & Diabetes Research Center
196 Richmond Street, Providence, RI 02903
Phone: 1-800-606-NWCR (6927)
http://www.nwcr.ws

USDA Center for Nutrition Policy and Promotion
3101 Park Center Drive
Alexandria, VA 22302-1594
http://www.choosemyplate.gov

Nutritional Information Sources:

ConsumerLab.com, LLC
333 Mamaroneck Avenue
White Plains, NY 10605
Main Number: 1-914-722-9149
Toll Free: 1-888-676-9929
http://www.consumerlab.com

Natural Medicines Comprehensive Database.
3120 W. March Lane, Stockton, CA 95219
Tel:(209) 472-2244
Fax:(209) 472-2249
http://naturaldatabase.therapeuticresearch.com

Tufts University Health & Nutrition Letter
P.O. Box 8517
Big Sandy, TX 757555-8517
1-800-274-7581.
http://www.tuftshealthletter.com

Deflame – Dr. David Seaman
200 2nd Ave. South, Unit #476
St Petersburg, FL 33701-4313
Phone: (855) DeFlame / (855) 333-5263
http://deflame.com

Vitasearch
Current Research in Nutrition and Integrative Medicine
http://www.vitasearch.com/

Exercise Resources:
ACSM – American College of Sports Medicine
401 West Michigan Street,
Indianapolis, IN 46202-3233
Ph:(317) 637-9200
Fax:(317) 634-7817
http://www.acsm.org

President's Council on Fitness, Sports & Nutrition
1101 Wootton Parkway, Suite 560
Rockville, MD 20852
Phone: 240-276-9567
Fax: 240-276-9860
www.fitness.gov

Medical Organizations:
American Academy of Anti-Aging Medicine
1801 N. Military Trail, Suite 200
Boca Raton, FL 33431

Toll-Free - US Only: (888) 997-0112
International: (561) 997-0112
Fax: (561) 997-0287
http://www.a4m.com

Dr. Joseph Mercola' website
http://www.mercola.com
1 (877) 985-2695 (Toll-Free)
Outside the United States:
1 (847) 252-4355

The Institute for Functional Medicine
Washington Office (Headquarters)
505 S. 336th Street Suite 500
Federal Way, WA 98003
Tel: 1.800.228.0622
Main office: 1.253.661.3010
Fax: 1.253.661.8310

The Institute for Functional Medicine
New Mexico Office
3600 Cerrillos Rd, Suite 712
Santa Fe, NM 87507
Tel: 1.505.471.9020
Fax: 1.505.424.3108
http://www.functionalmedicine.org/

Nutritional Companies:
Barn Dad Nutrition
150 Lake Drive, Suite 101
Wexford, PA 15090
Phone: Toll Free- 855.826.2429
Fax: 724.934.5707
http://www.barndadnutrition.com

MHP
21 Dwight Place
Fairfield, NJ, 07004
Toll Free: (888) 783-8844
Local: (973) 785-9055
http://mhpstrong.com

For Health Providers:
Anabolic Laboratories.
Manufacturing facilities are located
in Colorado Springs, Colorado &
Irvine, California.
1 800 344-4592
http://www.anaboliclabs.com

Apex Energetics
16592 Hale Ave.
Irvine, CA 92606
949-251-0152
Fax: 949-251-0153
http://www.apexenergetics.com

Strength and Conditioning:
National Strength and Conditioning Association
1885 Bob Johnson Dr.
Colorado Springs CO 80906
800-815-6826
http://nsca.com

Carini's House of Iron (2 Locations)
339 Changebridge Road
Pine Brook, NJ
Phone: 973-287-7824
20 Powers Drive
Paramus, NJ 07652
(973) 934-8432
http://carinishouseofiron.com

VIP Fitness Studio
1000 Wall Street West
Lyndhurst, NJ 07071
1-877-4- VIPFIT
http://www.vipfitnessstudio.com

Mixed Martial Arts/ Brazilian Jiu Jitsu
MMA University
153 Newark Pompton Turnpike
Little Falls, NJ 07424
Phone: 1 (973) 837-6248
http://themmauniversity.com

Dragon Spirit (2 locations)
718 Ridge Rd.
Lyndhurst, NJ 07071
(201)355-8236
550 Valley Brook Ave.
Lyndhurst, NJ 07071
(201)438-0350
http://www.dragonspiritmma.com

Team Carvalho Academy (3 locations US)
85-99 Hazel Street, 2nd Floor,
Paterson, New Jersey 07503
(973)553-5365

505 Route 10
Randolph, New Jersey 07869
(973)933-2620

156 West Passaic Street
Rochelle Park, NJ 07662
(201)562-8966
http://www.teamcarvalho.com

For MMA fighter management
MMAU Management
153 Newark Pompton Turnpike
Little Falls, NJ 07424
Phone: 1 (973) 837-6248

Kettlebell Training:
DragonDoor
1-800-899- 5111
http://www.dragondoor.com

Phil Ross/ American Eagle MMA & Kettlebells
500 Barnett Place
Ho-Ho-Kus, New Jersey 07423
Phone : (201) 612-1429
http://philross.com

Exercise Equipment
http://www.trxtraining.com
http://www.rackworkout.com
http://www.bodybyjake.com

Front Cover/ Photographer
Rachael Reis
Rachael Reis Photographyhttp://www.rachaelreisphotography.com

Contact Dr. Haley at 201-531-9400 or email haleychiro@yahoo.com for additional resources in your area.

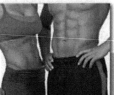

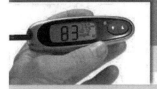
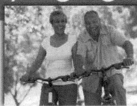